2

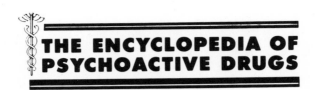

THE ENCYCLOPEDIA OF PSYCHOACTIVE DRUGS

SERIES 1

The Addictive Personality
Alcohol and Alcoholism
Alcohol Customs and Rituals
Alcohol Teenage Drinking
Amphetamines Danger in the Fast Lane
Barbiturates Sleeping Potion or Intoxicant?
Caffeine The Most Popular Stimulant
Cocaine A New Epidemic
Escape from Anxiety and Stress
Flowering Plants Magic in Bloom
Getting Help Treatments for Drug Abuse
Heroin The Street Narcotic
Inhalants The Toxic Fumes

LSD Visions or Nightmares?
Marijuana Its Effects on Mind & Body
Methadone Treatment for Addiction
Mushrooms Psychedelic Fungi
Nicotine An Old-Fashioned Addiction
Over-The-Counter Drugs Harmless or Hazardous?
PCP The Dangerous Angel
Prescription Narcotics The Addictive Painkillers
Quaaludes The Quest for Oblivion
Teenage Depression and Drugs
Treating Mental Illness
Valium and Other Tranquilizers

SERIES 2

Bad Trips
Brain Function
Case Histories
Celebrity Drug Use
Designer Drugs
The Downside of Drugs
Drinking, Driving, and Drugs
Drugs and Civilization
Drugs and Crime
Drugs and Diet
Drugs and Disease
Drugs and Emotion
Drugs and Pain
Drugs and Perception
Drugs and Pregnancy
Drugs and Sexual Behavior

Drugs and Sleep
Drugs and Sports
Drugs and the Arts
Drugs and the Brain
Drugs and the Family
Drugs and the Law
Drugs and Women
Drugs of the Future
Drugs Through the Ages
Drug Use Around the World
Legalization: A Debate
Mental Disturbances
Nutrition and the Brain
The Origins and Sources of Drugs
Substance Abuse: Prevention and Treatment
Who Uses Drugs?

EMOTIONS & THOUGHTS

GENERAL EDITOR
Professor Solomon H. Snyder, M.D.

*Distinguished Service Professor of
Neuroscience, Pharmacology, and Psychiatry at
The Johns Hopkins University School of Medicine*

•

ASSOCIATE EDITOR
Professor Barry L. Jacobs, Ph.D.

*Program in Neuroscience, Department of Psychology,
Princeton University*

•

SENIOR EDITORIAL CONSULTANT
Joann Rodgers

*Deputy Director, Office of Public Affairs at
The Johns Hopkins Medical Institutions*

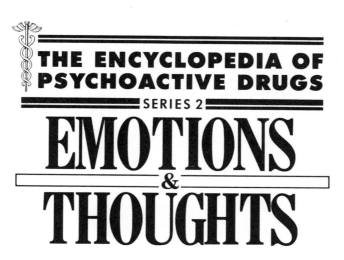

THE ENCYCLOPEDIA OF PSYCHOACTIVE DRUGS
SERIES 2
EMOTIONS & THOUGHTS

BRUCE FRIEDLAND

CHELSEA HOUSE PUBLISHERS
NEW YORK • NEW HAVEN • PHILADELPHIA

Chelsea House Publishers
EDITOR-IN-CHIEF: Nancy Toff
EXECUTIVE EDITOR: Remmel T. Nunn
MANAGING EDITOR: Karyn Gullen Browne
COPY CHIEF: Juliann Barbato
PICTURE EDITOR: Adrian G. Allen
ART DIRECTOR: Giannella Garrett
MANUFACTURING MANAGER: Gerald Levine

The Encyclopedia of Psychoactive Drugs
SENIOR EDITOR: Jane Larkin Crain

Staff for: EMOTIONS AND THOUGHTS
ASSOCIATE EDITOR: Paula Edelson
ASSISTANT EDITORS: Laura-Ann Dolce, James Cornelius
COPY EDITOR: Terrance Dolan
DEPUTY COPY CHIEF: Ellen Scordato
EDITORIAL ASSISTANT: Susan DeRosa
ASSOCIATE PICTURE RESEARCHER: Juliette Dickstein
PICTURE RESEARCHER: Nisa Rauschenberg
DESIGNER: Victoria Tomaselli
PRODUCTION COORDINATOR: Joseph Romano
COVER ILLUSTRATION: Samuel Bayer

First Printing

1   3   5   7   9   8   6   4   2

Library of Congress Cataloging in Publication Data

Friedland, Bruce.
    Emotions and Thoughts.

    (The Encyclopedia of psychoactive drugs. Series 2).
    Bibliography: p.
    Includes index.
    Summary: Discusses normal emotions and the thought process and how they
are directly affected by drugs.
    1. Psychotropic drugs—Juvenile literature. 2. Drug abuse—Psychological
aspects—Juvenile literature. 3. Emotions—Juvenile literature. 4. Thought and
thinking—Juvenile literature. [1. Emotions. 2. Thought and thinking. 3. Drug
abuse—Psychological aspects] I. Title.   II. Series.
RM315.F75   1987   616.86′3   88-9538

ISBN 1-55546-205-7

CONTENTS

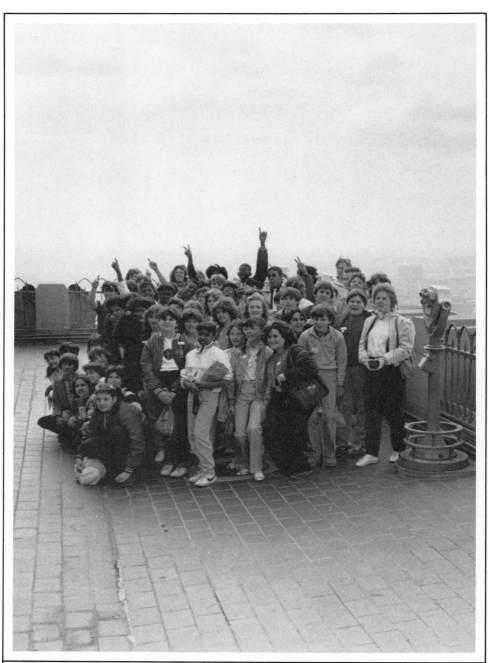

Every person is capable of experiencing a broad spectrum of emotions, including feelings of camaraderie. Drug use, however, can distort emotions and often leads to feelings of isolation.

FOREWORD

In the Mainstream
of American Life

One of the legacies of the social upheaval of the 1960s is that psychoactive drugs have become part of the mainstream of American life. Schools, homes, and communities cannot be "drug proofed." There is a demand for drugs — and the supply is plentiful. Social norms have changed and drugs are not only available—they are everywhere.

But where efforts to curtail the supply of drugs and outlaw their use have had tragically limited effects on demand, it may be that education has begun to stem the rising tide of drug abuse among young people and adults alike.

Over the past 25 years, as drugs have become an increasingly routine facet of contemporary life, a great many teenagers have adopted the notion that drug taking was somehow a right or a privilege or a necessity. They have done so, however, without understanding the consequences of drug use during the crucial years of adolescence.

The teenage years are few in the total life cycle, but critical in the maturation process. During these years adolescents face the difficult tasks of discovering their identity, clarifying their sexual roles, asserting their independence, learning to cope with authority, and searching for goals that will give their lives meaning.

Drugs rob adolescents of precious time, stamina, and health. They interrupt critical learning processes, sometimes forever. Teenagers who use drugs are likely to withdraw increasingly into themselves, to "cop out" at just the time when they most need to reach out and experience the world.

9

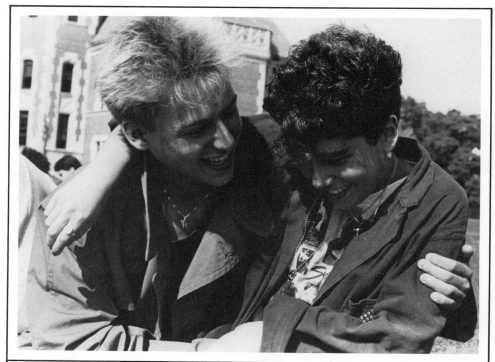

The feelings of mutual attraction and affection that people have for each other are often a source of pleasure but they can be quite deceptive when the use of psychoactive drugs is involved.

Fortunately, as a recent Gallup poll shows, young people are beginning to realize this, too. They themselves label drugs their most important problem. In the last few years, moreover, the climate of tolerance and ignorance surrounding drugs has been changing.

Adolescents as well as adults are becoming aware of mounting evidence that every race, ethnic group, and class is vulnerable to drug dependency.

Recent publicity about the cost and failure of drug rehabilitation efforts; dangerous drug use among pilots, air traffic controllers, star athletes, and Hollywood celebrities; and drug-related accidents, suicides, and violent crime have focused the public's attention on the need to wage an all-out war on drug abuse before it seriously undermines the fabric of society itself.

The anti-drug message is getting stronger and there is evidence that the message is beginning to get through to adults and teenagers alike.
war on drug abuse before it seriously undermines the fabric of society itself.

The anti-drug message is getting stronger and there is evidence that the message is beginning to get through to adults and teenagers alike.

The Encyclopedia of Psychoactive Drugs hopes to play a part in the national campaign now underway to educate young people about drugs. Series 1 provides clear and comprehensive discussions of common psychoactive substances, outlines their psychological and physiological effects on the mind and body, explains how they "hook" the user, and separates fact from myth in the complex issue of drug abuse.

Whereas Series 1 focuses on specific drugs, such as nicotine or cocaine, Series 2 confronts a broad range of both social and physiological phenomena. Each volume addresses the ramifications of drug use and abuse on some aspect of human experience: social, familial, cultural, historical, and physical. Separate volumes explore questions about the effects of drugs on brain chemistry and unborn children; the use and abuse of painkillers; the relationship between drugs and sexual behavior, sports, and the arts; drugs and disease; the role of drugs in history; and the sophisticated drugs now being developed in the laboratory that will profoundly change the future.

Each book in the series is fully illustrated and is tailored to the needs and interests of young readers. The more adolescents know about drugs and their role in society, the less likely they are to misuse them.

Joann Rodgers
Senior Editorial Consultant

FOWLERS AND WELLS,

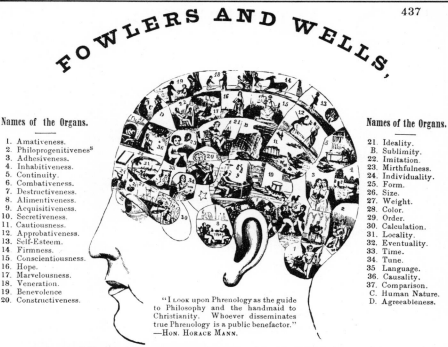

Names of the Organs.

1. Amativeness.
2. Philoprogenitiveness
3. Adhesiveness.
4. Inhabitiveness.
5. Continuity.
6. Combativeness.
7. Destructiveness.
8. Alimentiveness.
9. Acquisitiveness.
10. Secretiveness.
11. Cautiousness.
12. Approbativeness.
13. Self-Esteem.
14. Firmness.
15. Conscientiousness.
16. Hope.
17. Marvelousness.
18. Veneration.
19. Benevolence
20. Constructiveness.

Names of the Organs.

21. Ideality.
B. Sublimity.
22. Imitation.
23. Mirthfulness.
24. Individuality.
25. Form.
26. Size.
27. Weight.
28. Color.
29. Order.
30. Calculation.
31. Locality.
32. Eventuality.
33. Time.
34. Tune.
35. Language.
36. Causality.
37. Comparison.
C. Human Nature.
D. Agreeableness.

"I look upon Phrenology as the guide to Philosophy and the handmaid to Christianity. Whoever disseminates true Phrenology is a public benefactor." —Hon. Horace Mann.

PHRENOLOGISTS,

142 WASHINGTON ST., BOSTON,

308 BROADWAY, NEW YORK,

231 ARCH ST., PHILADELPHIA.

OUR CABINETS OR MUSEUMS

Contain Busts and Casts from the heads of the most distinguished men that ever lived; also Skulls, human and animal, from all quarters of the globe—including Egyptian Mummies, Pirates, Robbers, Murderers and Thieves; also numerous Paintings and Drawings of celebrated Individuals, living and dead. Strangers and citizens will find our Phrenological Rooms an agreeable place to visit.

PHRENOLOGICAL EXAMINATIONS

AND ADVICE, with Charts and full Written Descriptions of Character, given, when desired. These MENTAL portraits, as guides to self-culture, are invaluable.

THE UTILITY OF PHRENOLOGY.

Phrenology teaches us our natural capacities, our right and wrong tendencies, the most appropriate avocations, and directs us how to attain self-improvement, happiness, and success in life.

VALUABLE PUBLICATIONS.

Fowlers and Wells have all works on Phrenology, Physiology, Phonography, Hydropathy, and the Natural Sciences generally.

An advertisement for phrenologists, who believed that character was determined by the shape of the head. Today most scientists agree that character is shaped by environment and ancestry.

INTRODUCTION

The Gift of Wizardry
Use and Abuse

JACK H. MENDELSON, M.D.
NANCY K. MELLO, Ph.D.
Alcohol and Drug Abuse Research Center
Harvard Medical School—McLean Hospital

Dorothy to the Wizard:

"I think you are a very bad man," said Dorothy.
"Oh no, my dear; I'm really a very good man; but I'm a very bad Wizard."
—from THE WIZARD OF OZ

Man is endowed with the gift of wizardry, a talent for discovery and invention. The discovery and invention of substances that change the way we feel and behave are among man's special accomplishments, and, like so many other products of our wizardry, these substances have the capacity to harm as well as to help. Psychoactive drugs can cause profound changes in the chemistry of the brain and other vital organs, and although their legitimate use can relieve pain and cure disease, their abuse leads in a tragic number of cases to destruction.

Consider alcohol — available to all and yet regarded with intense ambivalence from biblical times to the present day. The use of alcoholic beverages dates back to our earliest ancestors. Alcohol use and misuse became associated with the worship of gods and demons. One of the most powerful Greek gods was Dionysus, lord of fruitfulness and god of wine. The Romans adopted Dionysus but changed his name to Bacchus. Festivals and holidays associated with Bacchus celebrated the harvest and the origins of life. Time has blurred the images of the Bacchanalian festival, but the theme of drunkenness as a major part of celebration has survived the pagan gods and remains a familiar part of modern society. The term "Bacchanalian Festival" conveys a more appealing image than "drunken orgy" or "pot party," but whatever the label, drinking alcohol is a form of drug use that results in addiction for millions.

The fact that many millions of other people can use alcohol in moderation does not mitigate the toll this drug takes on society as a whole. According to reliable estimates, one out of every ten Americans develops a serious alcohol-related problem sometime in his or her lifetime. In addition, automobile accidents caused by drunken drivers claim the lives of tens of thousands every year. Many of the victims are gifted young people, just starting out in adult life. Hospital emergency rooms abound with patients seeking help for alcohol-related injuries.

Who is to blame? Can we blame the many manufacturers who produce such an amazing variety of alcoholic beverages? Should we blame the educators who fail to explain the perils of intoxication, or so exaggerate the dangers of drinking that no one could possibly believe them? Are friends to blame — those peers who urge others to "drink more and faster," or the macho types who stress the importance of being able to "hold your liquor"? Casting blame, however, is hardly constructive, and pointing the finger is a fruitless way to deal with the problem. Alcoholism and drug abuse have few culprits but many victims. Accountability begins with each of us, every time we choose to use or misuse an intoxicating substance.

It is ironic that some of man's earliest medicines, derived from natural plant products, are used today to poison and to intoxicate. Relief from pain and suffering is one of society's many continuing goals. Over 3,000 years ago, the Therapeutic Papyrus of Thebes, one of our earliest written records, gave instructions for the use of opium in the treatment of pain. Opium, in the form of its major derivative, morphine, and similar compounds, such as heroin, have also been used by many to induce changes in mood and feeling. Another example of man's misuse of a natural substance is the coca leaf, which for centuries was used by the Indians of Peru to reduce fatigue and hunger. Its modern derivative, cocaine, has important medical use as a local anesthetic. Unfortunately, its increasing abuse in the 1980s clearly has reached epidemic proportions.

The purpose of this series is to explore in depth the psychological and behavioral effects that psychoactive drugs have on the individual, and also, to investigate the ways in which drug use influences the legal, economic, cultural, and even moral aspects of societies. The information presented here (and in other books in this series) is based on many clinical and laboratory studies and other observations by people from diverse walks of life.

Over the centuries, novelists, poets, and dramatists have provided us with many insights into the sometimes seductive but ultimately problematic aspects of alcohol and drug use. Physicians, lawyers, biologists, psychologists, and social scientists have contributed to a better understanding of the causes and consequences of using these substances. The authors in this series have attempted to gather and condense all the latest information about drug use and abuse. They have also described the sometimes wide gaps in our knowledge and have suggested some new ways to answer many difficult questions.

One such question, for example, is how do alcohol and drug problems get started? And what is the best way to treat them when they do? Not too many years ago, alcoholics and drug abusers were regarded as evil, immoral, or both. It is now recognized that these persons suffer from very complicated diseases involving deep psychological and social problems. To understand how the disease begins and progresses, it is necessary to understand the nature of the substance, the behavior of addicts, and the characteristics of the society or culture in which they live.

Although many of the social environments we live in are very similar, some of the most subtle differences can strongly influence our thinking and behavior. Where we live, go to school and work, whom we discuss things with — all influence our opinions about drug use and misuse. Yet we also share certain commonly accepted beliefs that outweigh any differences in our attitudes. The authors in this series have tried to identify and discuss the central, most crucial issues concerning drug use and misuse.

Despite the increasing sophistication of the chemical substances we create in the laboratory, we have a long way to go in our efforts to make these powerful drugs work for us rather than against us.

The volumes in this series address a wide range of timely questions. What influence has drug use had on the arts? Why do so many of today's celebrities and star athletes use drugs, and what is being done to solve this problem? What is the relationship between drugs and crime? What is the physiological basis for the power drugs can hold over us? These are but a few of the issues explored in this far-ranging series.

Educating people about the dangers of drugs can go a long way towards minimizing the desperate consequences of substance abuse for individuals and society as a whole. Luckily, human beings have the resources to solve even the most serious problems that beset them, once they make the commitment to do so. As one keen and sensitive observer, Dr. Lewis Thomas, has said,

> There is nothing at all absurd about the human condition. We matter. It seems to me a good guess, hazarded by a good many people who have thought about it, that we may be engaged in the formation of something like a mind for the life of this planet. If this is so, we are still at the most primitive stage, still fumbling with language and thinking, but infinitely capacitated for the future. Looked at this way, it is remarkable that we've come as far as we have in so short a period, really no time at all as geologists measure time. We are the newest, youngest, and the brightest thing around.

EMOTIONS & THOUGHTS

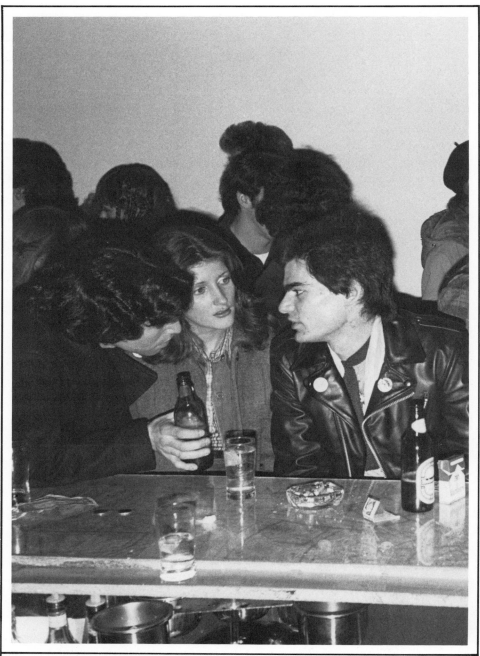

Although drinking alcohol in moderation can relieve tension — particularly in social situations — long-term use of the drug can result in severe emotional damage as well as addiction.

This book is part of a series of books that attempts to answer the many questions that students, parents, and teachers ask about drugs. Because there *are* so many questions, the topics of these books range from specific problems such as drinking and driving to the more general impact of drugs on society, the family, and the individual. This volume, *Emotions and Thoughts*, examines those aspects of mental life that are most directly affected by drug use.

Chapter 1, "What is Normal?" explores the spectrum of healthy emotional responses, and discusses the powerful and dangerous effects of drug use on the normal processes of emotion and thought. The goal of this chapter is to point out the difficulties of coping with the *normal* stresses of everyday life, and to warn of the dangers of retreating into drug use as a way of doing this. This leads us to the more specific discussions of healthy mental life that follow.

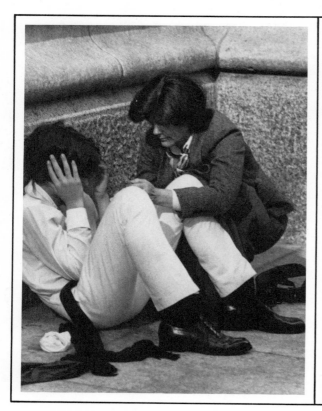

The nature of emotions is a mysterious area in the study of psychology, dependent on a complicated mixture of sensations, memories, drives, and habits.

Are you an optimist? A pessimist? Are you outgoing? Shy? Your personality is the topic of Chapter 2, which begins by asking whether it can be changed. The answer, of course, is that it can — but the degree to which one's personality can be changed, and the degree to which it may be inherited, is a complex question that has not been fully answered. In this chapter we explore several attempts to answer it, and we also examine some ideas about personality put forward by such prominent theorists as Sigmund Freud, Abraham Maslow, and B. F. Skinner. Examining these theories of personality types can help us put our own personalities into perspective.

Next we look at the nature of emotions. This is still a mysterious area in the study of psychology, but examining such specific emotions as anxiety can teach us a great deal about the physiological and cognitive factors that blend together to create our emotional responses to our environment.

Emotions and thoughts, however, do not alone determine our behavior; they rest upon a complicated mixture of sensations, memories, drives, and habits. In the final chapters of this book we examine psychological and physiological processes that underlie consciousness and sexuality, and that enable us to remember and learn. These processes are as fragile as they are complex, and the effects of drug use are nowhere more apparent than here.

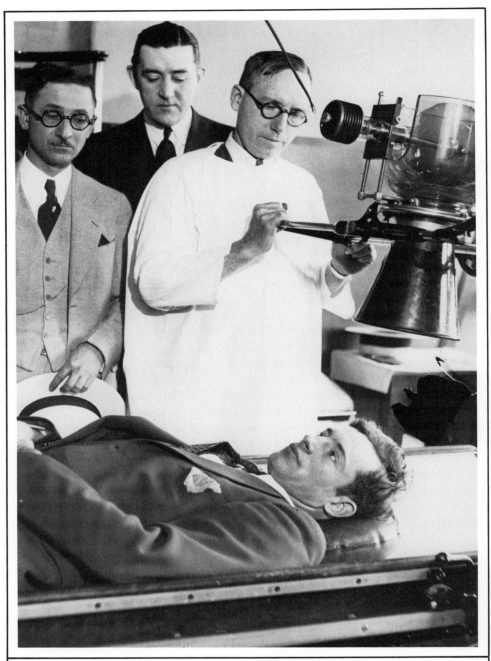

In 1931, a doctor analyzes an accused murderer's sanity by x-raying his skull. Modern tests are far more sophisticated, but experts still disagree about the physiological basis of behavior.

CHAPTER 1

WHAT IS NORMAL?

Is there such a thing as normal? One task of recent clinical studies on emotion is to try to define what, if anything, is normal human emotional behavior. Obviously, each person is different, but do most people generally exhibit certain types of behavior in certain situations? Can thought patterns be predicted on the basis of past observation? The complexity of human personality is vast, perhaps so vast that to call anyone "normal" is unfair to that person as well as to every other person; the complexity of human feelings and emotions cannot be so neatly dissected and understood.

Although psychologists regularly diagnose abnormal behaviors such as anxiety, depression, and schizophrenia, making sense of the wide range of so-called normal emotional behavior, and the factors that influence it, is a far different matter. Research goes on in an effort to find, if not what is "normal," then at least what is abnormal enough to be called emotionally unhealthy behavior.

Emotional Contraries

Consider the emotion of anger. Every person knows what it is to be angry — angry at himself or herself, at others, at the world. In its milder forms, anger can lead to frustration, confrontation, and bitterness. In more extreme cases, it can es-

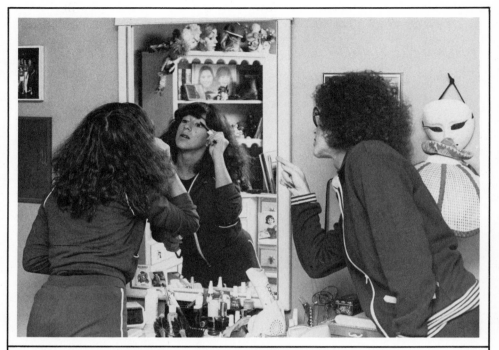

A mother-daughter confrontation. Anger and aggression are often perceived as unhealthy and unattractive behaviors, but both are common and universal human personality traits.

calate into full-blown rage. Think of how much senseless violence might be eliminated from society if anger were simply erased from our emotional repertoire. Should the emotion of anger, then, be considered abnormal because of its destructive potential, or normal because of its universality?

Take another example. It is widely perceived today that aggression, a powerful human behavior, is not only emotionally unhealthy but unattractive as a personality trait. Yet sports that unabashedly glorify aggression, such as football and boxing, have mass appeal; meanwhile, war is continuously fought at various points on the globe. Most of the people engaged in these supposedly unhealthy pursuits are considered well adjusted.

Similarly, wouldn't most people agree that fear is an unpleasant and unwanted emotion? To walk down a dark street alone at night and hear footsteps suddenly coming up from behind is to know just how unpleasant fear can be. Still, people of all ages and occupations sometimes go out of their way to have fear-inducing experiences, whether it be at horror films, on the roller coaster at the fair, or perhaps while rock climbing.

On the positive end of the emotional spectrum is love. Yet love is perhaps the strongest and most unpredictable human feeling of all. People have waged wars for the sake of love, and kings have given up kingdoms for it. Poets, writers, and artists have pondered love's power, sometimes praising and sometimes bemoaning it. Journalist and pundit H. L. Mencken wrote, "Love is like war; easy to begin but very hard to stop." Love for the individual may be like war for a nation: almost unavoidable, potentially liberating, possibly devastating. Many people will kill for love of their country or religion, yet soldiers are not considered insane. These are just examples of how two supposedly contrary emotions, love and aggression, can overlap.

The Spectrum of Normality

With all these paradoxes, is it possible to determine what constitutes normal emotional behavior? Furthermore, what distinguishes normal from abnormal behavior and more serious mental disorders?

By definition, a thing is normal if it conforms to a standard or a typical pattern. As we have seen, however, standards and patterns of feelings and emotions change frequently — there are so many variables, it would be foolhardy to say that aggression is always unhealthy or that fear is always unpleasant or that love is always wonderful.

How, for example, would you classify the behavior of an otherwise thoughtful, intelligent woman who smokes cigarettes during pregnancy? Although she is aware of the documented health risks to herself and her unborn baby, she continues to smoke. Can this be considered emotionally normal? Virtually all studies have found that nicotine, the acting drug in cigarettes, promotes lung cancer and other respiratory diseases such as chronic bronchitis and emphysema. Why do smokers go on smoking? Why, for that matter, do people snort cocaine or inject heroin or ingest any other drug that could severely damage their bodies or disrupt their lives?

There is no simple answer to those questions. In many ways, feelings and emotions are like the weather, and even the most mentally healthy people have their bright days and their stormy ones. Rigid standards for normal feelings and emotions do not work, because each mind encompasses a vast spectrum of emotional behavior.

Thus, the behavior of the football fanatic and the horror show enthusiast can be seen as normal even though feelings of aggression and fear are not generally considered emotionally healthy. And smokers, whose behavior could literally kill them, cannot simply be dismissed as insane.

Ironic as it may seem, the spectrum of normality takes into account abnormal behavior. It is not only possible but highly probable that normal individuals will occasionally engage in maladaptive behavior, that is, behavior that deviates from the social norm. By itself, however, such behavior (smoking, for instance) does not preclude or necessarily inhibit overall successful functioning in society.

Sometimes, however, the intensity of our emotions can be overwhelming, even to the point of mimicking serious mental disorders such as depression, acute anxiety, and paranoia. Yet even these strong emotions can fall within the bounds of normality so long as they do not substantially or consistently disrupt mental or physical processes or cause a loss of self-control.

Anger turned to rage, for example, is certainly maladaptive behavior, yet it can still fall within the vast framework of normality. No matter how angry a person may become, most people manage to control the manner in which they act upon their feelings. But when an individual's rage boils over into violence, it signals a loss of mental and physical control. Such behavior, if accompanied by a significant disruption or distortion of mental and physical processes, can result in a severe deviation from the social norm and even a total break with reality.

Still, isolated incidents of intense, even overwhelming emotion are not by themselves signs of mental illness. In fact, it is likely that every normal human being will experience many intense emotions in the course of his or her lifetime:

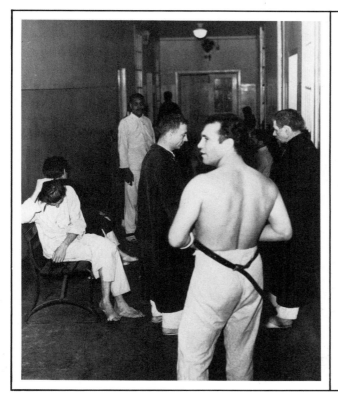

A 1949 photograph captures the grimness of a ward in a mental hospital. Advances in the methods of treating mental illness have dramatically improved the conditions in such hospitals.

During a time of crisis like a house fire or an automobile accident; attending the funeral of a loved one; in a combat situation; or perhaps during more joyful occasions like marriage and childbirth.

The most important factor to keep in mind regarding normal behavior is that no person is emotionally perfect. The various stresses of living in an imperfect world often create situations in which maladaptive and occasionally abnormal emotional responses are to be expected.

Coping

Many psychologists believe that the people with the best mental health are those who can easily adjust to the onslaught of change in the world and the consequent disruption of their own feelings. Ordinarily, most human beings manage this feat exceedingly well.

We all experience, and cope with, a wide range of feelings and emotions every day of our lives: fear, happiness, sadness, disappointment, disgust, anger, boredom, excitement. Think, for a moment, of the different feelings you have experienced since waking up this morning. Experiencing and coping with an assortment of emotions of varying intensity is so common to everyday life that often we may not even realize we are doing it. In a study conducted by psychologist James Averill, college students and adults were asked to keep a record of every time they became annoyed or angry. The results showed that some participants in the study became mildly to moderately angry from several times a week to several times a day. Imagine how much time it would take to record *all* the feelings and emotions you experience over the course of one week.

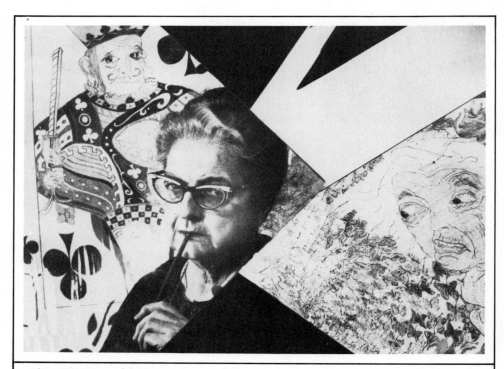

This 71-year-old woman was able to cure her depression by learning to draw. Human beings have remarkable coping mechanisms that enable them to deal with a wide range of emotions.

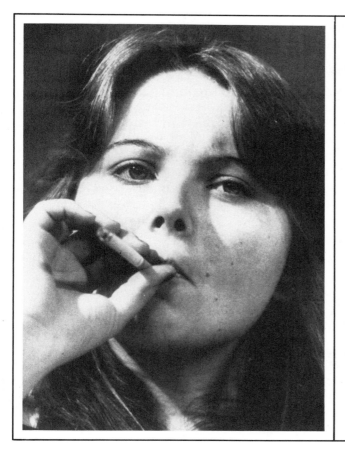

Many adolescents in American society feel peer pressure to experiment with both legal and illegal drugs.

Some researchers believe that man's original emotions were both early warning signals against attack and preparation for defense. When primitive man perceived a stressful or threatening situation, certain physiological, or bodily, responses followed that energized the individual for what has been termed *fight or flight*.

Although we are no longer faced with the same survival problems as our ancestors, modern man still experiences a variety of stresses and emotionally threatening situations. And our bodies still react. When embarrassed we blush; when angered our eyes narrow and our teeth clench; when frightened our pulse quickens and we turn pale or begin to sweat. Conversely, when we are happy we smile and laugh. If we are extremely happy, we may cry.

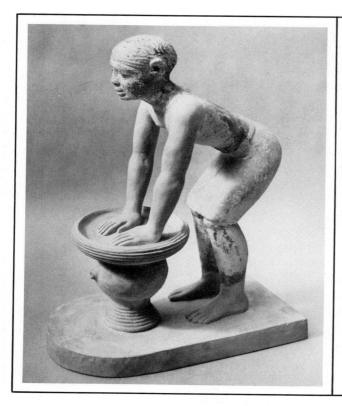

A 3rd-century, B.C.E., statue of a beer maker. The use of drugs is as old as civilization, but the percentage of people who use chemical substances to help them cope with emotional traumas has increased dramatically in the late 20th century.

Coping with Drugs

Over the last 30 years, individuals have increasingly used the aid of chemical substances to cope with emotional turbulence. What began as a great boon to humanity in the form of new medicine has turned slowly toward an equally great disaster: widespread addiction to new chemical derivatives, and the recreational use of powerful drugs such as LSD, heroin, and PCP.

The connection between drug use and human emotion and thought is a slippery one. So advanced is the state of laboratory chemistry and our comprehension of how the brain works, that for each emotion there may well be a corresponding drug to quell or prolong it.

Despite the enormous number of emotions that humans are able to feel, some psychologists theorize that every one of them is rooted in one of two primary sensations: distress or delight. Life is the quest to capture as much of the latter as possible, and if drugs help one find that state, albeit temporarily, then many people will take them.

In American society, there is a degree of social pressure to use certain drugs (legal and illegal) "recreationally" — to create a sensation of pleasure. This pressure finds an audience among people from all walks of life, especially among those who feel trapped or are otherwise unhappy, and that includes a great many teenagers. The emotional turmoil of adolescence is for most people the roughest they will ever know, and drug use can be a quick way out. But drug use can also exacerbate an already difficult situation.

In exploring some of what is known about human emotional content and our sensory, perceptual, and cognitive systems, we can also apply some of what is known or theorized about the influence of various drugs on those emotions and thoughts. Drug abuse, including the abuse of legal drugs, may be a "normal" way for some people to cope, but the overall danger is leading most experts today to recommend otherwise.

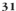

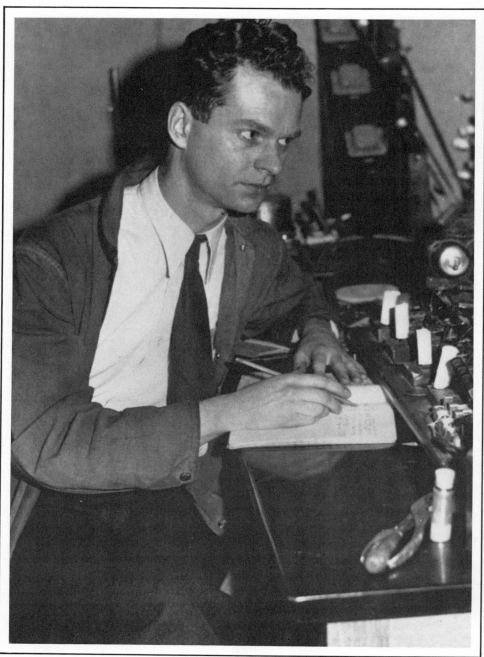

The behavioral psychologist B. F. Skinner, shown here in 1933, believes that human behavior is shaped primarily by forces in the environment, rather than by hereditary factors.

CHAPTER 2

PERSONALITY

We all know people whose warmth, humor, and compassion make them attractive as friends and companions. We also know people who seem unfriendly, irritable, obnoxiously loud, or painfully shy. Although we casually label such individuals as having a "good" or "bad" personality, to psychologists, personality is not simply what makes an individual fun or boring but is rather the complex interaction of many elements that combine to shape the distinctive ways in which we relate to the world.

Personality can be thought of as the sum total of an individual's behavioral traits. To adequately understand personality, then, all aspects of human behavior must be considered. Emotion, perception, cognition, the use of language: All of these play an integral role in determining why we are the way we are.

One of the most basic questions is this: To what extent do individuals inherit personality from their parents, and to what extent do they acquire it as learned behavior from their environment? This is called the *nature-nurture* question, and it has fascinated philosophers, scientists, and scholars for centuries.

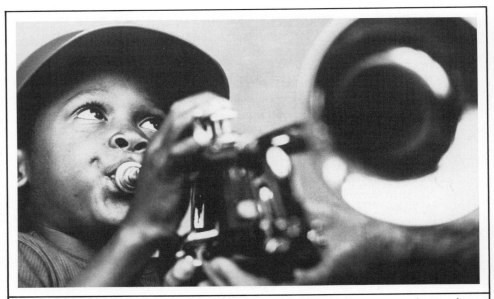

Experts disagree as to whether musical and other talents are inherited or if they can be taught by conditioning techniques.

Although today it is believed that *both* heredity and environment help shape personality, earlier psychologists were drawn to either one side of the issue or the other. Those scientists who believed behavior was a function of heredity pointed to the various species of animals who exhibited instinctive, or unlearned, behavior. Certain birds, for instance, instinctively know how to build nests even when they are raised in isolation and have never seen a nest being built. Numerous other animals, with no practice or observation, know how to hunt, mate, and defend themselves against predators.

Researchers speculated that heredity was responsible for such instinctive behavior. They further speculated that human behavior was based on similar instincts. Traits like intelligence, mood, and aggression, they reasoned, had nothing to do with environmental factors.

That theory was opposed by a group of scientists known as *behaviorists*, who agreed that human behavior was the result of environmental learning only. John Watson, founder of the behaviorist school, based this claim on a more fundamental argument about the nature of psychology itself. He believed that psychology should only concern itself with what can be observed or scientifically measured, and that because inherited traits *cannot* be observed or measured, they cannot be postulated even to exist, much less considered responsible for behavior. Behaviorists also believe that almost any kind of behavior can be taught through various conditioning techniques, and indeed, conditioning has proven to be a powerful tool in the shaping of human personality.

Although modern science understands that both nature and nurture play a significant role in shaping personality, the issue of how great a role each plays is still very much undecided.

The Study of Twins

Jim Springer and Jim Lewis are very special brothers, especially with regard to the issue of nature-nurture. It is only a coincidence that they share the same first name, but it is no coincidence at all that they have different last names, for these

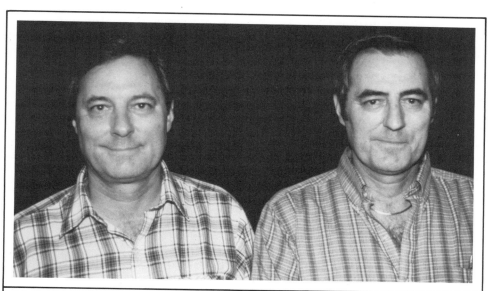

Though separated at birth, twins Jim Springer and Jim Lewis still exhibited similar personality characteristics. Such cases suggest that some traits are more heritable than scientists once believed.

identical twins were separated at birth and not reunited until decades later. Because they are identical twins and therefore share precisely the same genetic makeup, the brothers offer researchers a unique insight into the factors that influence personality.

The Jim twins are part of an extensive study begun in 1979 at the University of Minnesota, which was designed to compare the behavior of identical twins who had been reared apart. By studying pairs of people whose genetic makeup was identical but whose environment had been totally different, researchers hoped to learn something about the degree to which traits and characteristics can be passed on genetically.

In addition to answering some 15,000 questions concerning their lives and behavior patterns, all twins were given an exhaustive battery of mental and physical tests. The results of X-rays, electrocardiograms, videotapes, and interviews, among other things, will eventually be reduced to statistical data, which will then be analyzed to see how closely the behavior of twins reared apart match.

Although much of the data has yet to be collected and analyzed, results of the Minnesota twin study thus far have been fascinating. For example, the Jim twins, though reared apart, had extremely similar personalities. They both had the habit of biting their nails, and both developed migraine headaches at the same age. Both worked at the same occupation, smoked the same brand of cigarette, drove the same kind of car, and enjoyed the same hobby of woodworking.

The study also found that identical twins reared apart seem to have similar immune systems. In many cases, the onset of disease occurred at the same time in each twin, as was the case with the Jim twins' migraine headaches. The research also shows that identical twins reared apart have similar cardiac and respiratory systems as well as brain-wave patterns.

These similarities lead to the obvious conclusion that traits and characteristics are far more heritable (capable of being inherited) than once believed. If that is indeed the case, then traits such as intelligence and creativity might also be determined by our genetic blueprints, much the same way that height and eye color are. However, disorders such as obesity or alcoholism might also be more hereditary than once believed.

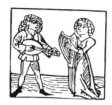

SANGUINE

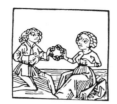

MELANCHOLIC

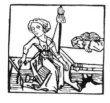

PHLEGMATIC

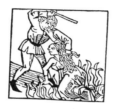

CHOLERIC

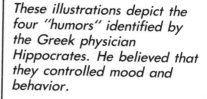

These illustrations depict the four "humors" identified by the Greek physician Hippocrates. He believed that they controlled mood and behavior.

Researchers are quick to point out that heritability alone does not guarantee a set behavior. Even though a person has been endowed with the heritable trait of musical ability, for example, he or she may never develop musical talent without the proper environmental influences — such as music teachers, availability of instruments, positive reinforcement from parents, etc. In short, both nature *and* nurture appear to play a role in the shaping of human behavior.

Theories of Personality

Studying identical twins reared apart will undoubtedly further our understanding of how personality is shaped, but it seems unlikely that any research will soon be able to identify exactly what percentage of behavior is heritable and what percent is attributable to environment. In the absence of such absolutes, psychologists have to rely instead on personality theories.

Such theories are certainly not new. As early as the 5th century B.C., the Greek physician Hippocrates theorized that people's moods were controlled by fluids in the body that he called "humors." Hippocrates believed the body contained four such humors: blood, phlegm, black bile, and yellow bile. If any one particular humor was dominant in a person, that humor was thought to dictate personality.

A person with excessive blood, for example, was characterized as sanguine — cheerful, passionate, and hot-blooded. Too much phlegm was thought to cause listlessness and slothfulness. A predominance of black bile signaled melancholia, or gloominess and pessimism. And a person with an excess of yellow bile was considered choleric — irritable, nervous, and ill-tempered.

Although the theory of the four humors was later discarded, people have been categorizing personality in one way or another ever since.

The Psychoanalytic Approach

One of the most influential theories of personality was put forward in the late 19th century by Sigmund Freud (1856–1939), and in many ways society is still feeling its

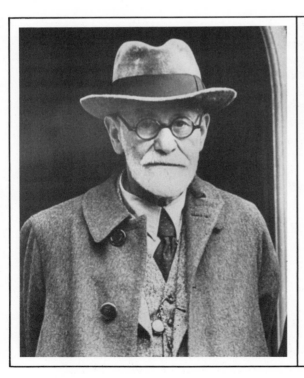

Sigmund Freud, the Viennese originator of psychoanalysis, theorized that human personality is determined by the interactions of three forces, which he called the id, ego, and superego.

effects. We have all heard, and probably used, terms like *ego* and *id*, *defense mechanism*, *fixation*, *psychoanalysis*, and *Freudian slip*.

Freud's theory, from which these terms derive, was essentially an outgrowth of his work with emotionally disturbed patients. Freud believed that physical and mental disorders, called "hysterical" disorders at the time, were caused by unconscious and unresolved sexual conflicts that usually originated in early childhood.

Freud's psychoanalytic theory was regarded as radical in its day because its underpinnings were based on the aggressive sexual nature of human beings and also because the idea of the unconscious — where strong motives and emotions dwelled without the individual being aware of them — had never been considered before by the prevailing scientific community.

In his patients, Freud attempted to liberate these unconscious feelings and bring them into the open, or conscious, mind, through a method of treatment called *psychoanalysis*. In this treatment, patients were often asked to discuss early childhood experiences and dreams, and to *free-associate*, which means to say whatever comes into one's mind when the therapist says a particular word.

Based on his discoveries from psychoanalysis, Freud was able to theorize not only about his emotionally disturbed patients but about the normal workings of the human psyche as well. Basically, he believed that human personality consists of three elements or forces: the id, ego, and superego.

The id is an impulsive, highly charged sexual force that seeks pleasure through any means. Unswerving in its demand for gratification, the id is often referred to as the *pleasure principle*. The ego, conversely, is known as the *reality principle*. The ego is how we perceive ourselves in relation to the world around us, when we view ourselves as logically thinking entities who understand both what society expects and the consequences of inappropriate behavior. Though to some extent the ego strives to satisfy the id, it more often acts as a moderator. The ego is the reason that, if we are hungry, for instance, we do not simply satisfy that hunger by taking food from someone else's plate.

The ego must also deal with the *superego*, the third element of Freud's personality model. In a way, the superego

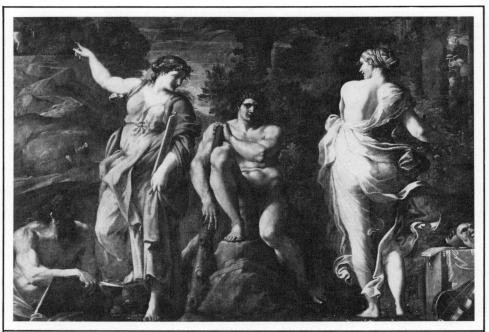

The Choice of Hercules *by Annibale Carracci can be thought of as an illustration of the ego's (Hercules') choice between the reflexes of the id (right) and the stern commands of the superego (left).*

represents social morals and standards. It is like a conscience. Where the id is sexual, impulsive, and demanding, the superego is ethical, demanding correct behavior and threatening punishment for anything that falls short of its expectations.

The constant, battling interplay of id, ego, and superego is much like the cartoon of the perplexed individual trying to decide if he should undertake some naughty behavior. There is a pitchfork-carrying devil sitting on his right shoulder, urging him to go ahead. On his left shoulder, an angel with a halo sternly cautions to hold back. Caught in the middle is the befuddled individual. According to Freud, the devil is the id, the angel is the superego, and the individual, trying to please both masters, is the ego.

The foundation of Freud's personality theory, then, is that we are constantly at odds with our inner selves, trying to resolve sexual conflicts and aggressive desires.

Humanistic Theories of Personality

In contrast to the Freudian model are the humanistic theories of personality. Whereas Freud's theory revolves around a ruthless, pleasure-seeking id, the humanists believe that man's core is basically desirous of peace, love, and harmony. Humanists believe in the idea of *self-actualization*, a concept developed by psychologist Abraham Maslow (1908–70).

As a counterpoint to Freudian theory, Maslow's belief is that human beings are innately good, and because of this they instinctively seek the good in themselves and others. However, such greater goals as love and fulfillment can only be achieved once the individual has satisfied certain basic needs. Maslow categorized a hierarchy of these needs in his personality model.

The primary need is physiological, the basic instinct for survival. We all must have food and water, and we all, according to Maslow, have the desire to reproduce, to continue

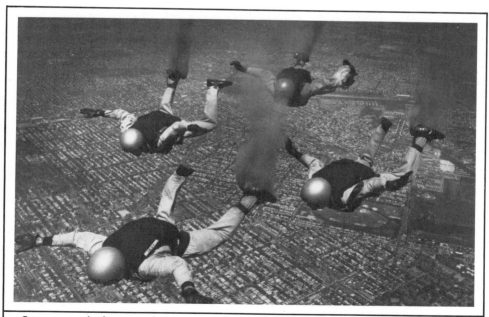

Some psychologists classify people according to personality types. The so-called thrill seeker, for example, is a person who enjoys a challenge or dare — such as skydiving — for its own sake.

the species. The next need in the hierarchy is safety. Human beings must have adequate shelter and a sense of order or stability to feel truly safe.

Once these needs are met, a person can turn his or her attention to higher levels of feeling. These Maslow classified as belongingness and love, self-esteem, and finally, at the highest level, self-actualization, which he described as self-fulfillment.

In his book *Toward a Psychology of Being*, Maslow writes of man's basic core of goodness: "This inner nature, as much as we know of it so far, seems not to be intrinsically or primarily or necessarily evil. . . . Human nature is not nearly as bad as it has been thought to be. . . ."

"It is as if Freud supplied to us the sick half of psychology and we must now fill it out with the healthy half. Perhaps this health psychology will give us more possibility for controlling and improving our lives and for making ourselves better people. Perhaps this will be more fruitful than asking 'how to get unsick.' "

Putting Theories to the Test

Unfortunately, despite its appeal to many people, there is no way to prove Maslow's theory. Like Freud's psychoanalytic theory, it offers no measurable, objective data, and to many scientists this failure is seen as a fatal flaw. The need for quantifiable data — that is, data to which statistical analysis can be applied — has led many psychologists away from both Freudian and humanistic theories and toward a theory called *behaviorism.*

The most famous of the modern day behaviorists is Harvard psychologist B. F. Skinner (1904–). His theory, radical behaviorism, suggests that human behavior is controlled exclusively by events in the environment. In fact, Skinner does not even see the need for a general theory of personality.

Skinner acknowledges the existence of inner thoughts and feelings, but in his model, these inner feelings are simply the by-products of external events. Behavior is either punished or rewarded based on learned experience. In other words, through learning, we constantly adjust our behavior to fit the situation. This would explain why a bully acts tough around those who are smaller than he is, and acts meek around those who are bigger. Skinner called this phenomenon *situation-specific* behavior.

There appears to be some validity to the theory, for behavior modification techniques are often used successfully to treat maladaptive behavior. Basically, by rewarding appropriate behavior with positive reinforcement and punishing inappropriate behavior with negative reinforcement, behavior can indeed be changed. Therapies to help people quit smoking and lose weight often use behavior modification techniques successfully.

Interestingly, these same techniques have been successfully used to treat alcoholism, although research indicates a substantial heritability factor between parents who are alcoholics and their children. In one study of twins, researchers found that adopted children who had been fathered by alcoholics were four times more likely to develop the disease later in life than were other adopted children whose fathers had not been alcoholics. Learning can overcome the heritability factor in many cases, but it can only go so far.

Personality Types

Through observation, psychologists have come to recognize a number of different personality types, each exhibiting certain specific traits, some of which are very healthy. Well-adjusted people, for example, are characterized by their ability to cope with a variety of emotional circumstances; a self-actualizing person, to use Maslow's term, continually strives for love, self-esteem, and fulfillment. Many personality types are not so positive, even though they fall well within the range of what psychologists call "normal." An individual with a compulsive personality, for example, is often absorbed in irrelevant details. A perfectionist by nature, the compulsive type is seldom spontaneous and is often serious to the point of boorishness.

A person with a passive-aggressive personality expresses resentment toward other people in an unusual way: He or she will act out aggression through inaction — stubbornness or procrastination, for instance. The passive-aggressive is almost always a pessimist.

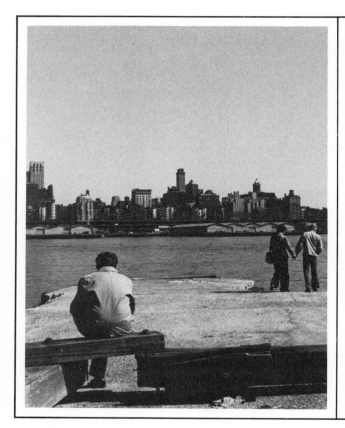

People with schizoid personalities are not actually schizophrenic, but are usually loners who are unable to form close relationships with others and seem on the fringe of society.

Other examples of *maladaptive personality types*:

•Schizoid: A loner, unable or unwilling to form close relationships with others, often absentminded and withdrawn from normal social endeavors. While not actually schizophrenic, a person with a schizoid personality often seems on the fringe of everyday reality.

•Histrionic: A very excitable person who seems to make mountains out of molehills. The histrionic type has a very large ego and places great demands on others for attention.

•Dependent: This personality type lacks self-confidence and almost always lets other people take control of the situation. A dependent person feels helpless but does not wish to be self-reliant.

•Avoidant: People with avoidant personalities are so fearful of rejection they generally avoid close relationships unless they are sure of success. They often feel inferior to others and are painfully sensitive to almost any kind of criticism.

Although these characteristics are often used to categorize serious personality disorders, it is normal to recognize several of these traits in healthy people — and in ourselves. At times, every person feels inferior, overly sensitive to criticism, compulsive, or afraid of rejection. These traits are only threatening if they begin to dominate a person's other, healthier traits and affect his or her ability to cope with reality. In the majority of cases, maladaptive personality traits represent only minor character flaws that may surface during stressful or other extreme emotional conditions.

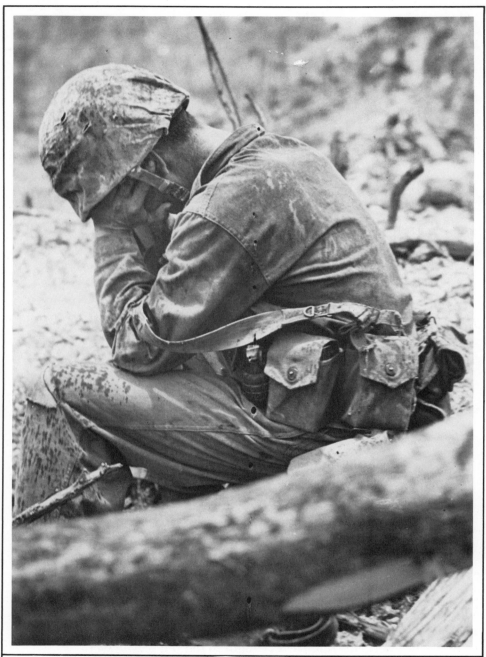

Emotions are present not only in crisis situations, such as battles, but in every aspect of daily living. The range of these feelings is wide, and their biological causes largely unknown.

CHAPTER 3

THE NATURE OF EMOTION

We were all strapped into the seats of the Chinook, fifty of us, and something, someone was hitting it from the outside with an enormous hammer. How do they do that? I thought, we're a thousand feet in the air! But it had to be that, over and over, shaking the helicopter, making it dip and turn in a horrible out-of-control motion that took me in the stomach. I had to laugh, it was so exciting, it was the thing I had wanted, almost what I had wanted except for the wrenching, resonant metal-echo; I could hear it even above the noise of the rotor blades. And they were going to fix that, I knew they would make it stop. They had to, it was going to make me sick.

They were all replacements going in to mop up after the big battles on Hills 875 and 876, the battles that had already taken on the names of one great battle, the battle of Dak To. And I was new, brand new, three days in-country, embarrassed about my boots because they were so new. And across from me ten feet away, a boy tried to jump out of the straps and then jerked forward and hung there, his rifle barrel caught in the red plastic webbing of the seat back. As the chopper rose again and turned, his weight went back hard against the webbing and a dark spot the size of a baby's hand showed in the center of his fatigue jacket. And it

grew — I knew what it was, but not really — it got up to his armpits and then started down his sleeves and up over his shoulders at the same time. It went all across his waist and down his legs, covering the canvas on his boots until they were dark like everything else he wore, and it was running in slow, heavy drops off his fingertips. I thought I could hear the drops hitting the metal strip on the chopper floor. Hey! ... Oh, but this isn't anything at all, it's not real, it's just some *thing* they're going through that isn't real. One of the door gunners was heaped up on the floor like a cloth dummy. His hand had the bloody raw look of a pound of liver fresh from the butcher paper. We touched down on the same [landing zone] we had just left a few minutes before, but I didn't know it until one of the guys shook my shoulder, and then I couldn't stand up. All I could feel of my legs was their shaking, and the guy thought I'd been hit and helped me up. The chopper had taken eight hits, there was shattered plastic all over the floor, a dying pilot up front, the boy was hanging forward in the straps again, he was dead, but not (I knew) really dead. ...
— From *Dispatches,* by Michael Herr

War correspondent Michael Herr had been in Vietnam for only three days and was anxious to see action when he had the above experience. So strong was his emotional reaction to witnessing a young man die that he denied the reality of what he had seen.

In the face of overwhelming emotion, denial is not an uncommon response. Just as a deer will freeze in the headlights of an oncoming car, people may also be immobilized, mentally and physically, in the face of crisis.

Emotions, however, are not present just during crisis situations but in every aspect of daily living. How did you feel, for example, reading Herr's passage above? When it became apparent that the writer was seeing the death of a young soldier, what emotions did you experience? Were you saddened, shocked, disgusted? Or were you fascinated by the power of the words? If so, did that fascination make you feel at all uneasy?

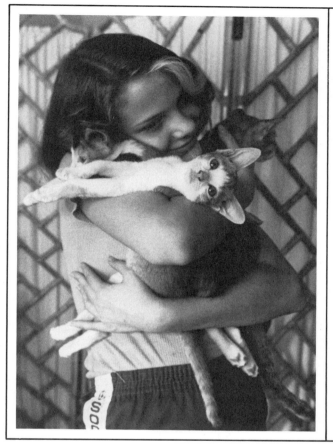

Emotions such as affection can vary greatly according to the situation. For example, love for a human and love for a cat are not necessarily the same feeling.

The range of normal emotions is diverse and encompasses a vast spectrum of feelings and behavior. You were probably not alone if you felt a sense of morbid fascination at Herr's vivid description of the helicopter attack. But why is that so? What, precisely, are emotions made of? What causes them to occur? Does everyone experience the same ones?

The Mystery of Emotion

Unfortunately, questions about the nature of emotion cannot be answered in absolute terms. Because emotional responses are largely internal, they are difficult to study. Like personality, much of what psychologists believe about emotion is based on theory.

Jean-Paul Sartre (1905–80), one of this century's great philosophers, believed that psychology, or any explanation of our emotions, can only be a collection of miscellaneous facts. As far as it is a science, he believed, psychology can assemble knowledge first about bodily reactions and then, perhaps, about behavior. But from there it tries to build a theory about the overall state of consciousness, which includes emotions. "The psychic facts we meet," he wrote, "are never the first ones. They are . . . man's reactions against the world." Getting to the essence of man's emotional makeup by assembling these various facts, then, is impossible; but that, in Sartre's view, is all the psychologist can hope to do.

An analogy might be the alphabet and Shakespeare's play *King Lear*: Merely knowing all the words the poet used does not reveal the pattern of how he used them, what each one means in its context, or how to predict what Lear might do next. Merely knowing the signs of each emotion does not reveal what causes them or what they mean in each situation.

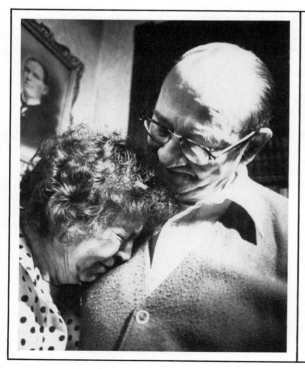

This couple has just found out that their son, who was held hostage in Iran, has been freed. One of the anomalies of human emotions is that tears are a sign of extreme happiness as well as of sorrow.

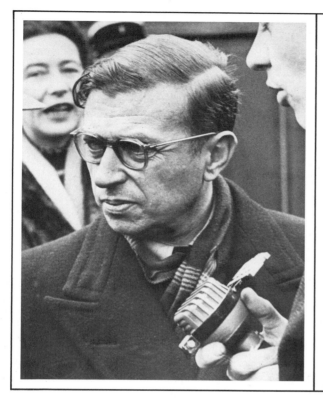

The philosopher Jean-Paul Sartre believed that each person's emotional makeup is so complex that devising a general theory of human behavior is impossible.

But even this comparison does not do justice to human emotion, for every individual is far more complex than a great work of literature.

Sartre's skepticism is not shared by all, especially in light of the great advances in neurological science made in the last 25 years. But he may be right at least in believing that the next step up the ladder, after observing emotions, is understanding behavior, and that that step will always be partially futile. Because everybody reacts differently, in his or her own way, it is difficult to predict or prove much about behavior. The brain can be measured; the mind cannot.

For example, being turned down for a job or for a date happens to everyone, but the reactions to that situation may range from dejection and sadness to anger or rage and the desire for revenge to anticipation of the next challenge. Many people could feel each of those things. For all of the data scientists might ever collect about the brain's role in emotions, the outside world as the mind perceives it involves too many variables to be measured.

Emotion versus Reason

Charles Darwin, whose theory of evolution rocked the scientific community in the 19th century, believed that many of our emotional expressions are not only universal but evolved from primitive man. Darwin found similarities in the expression of humans and lower animals. Wolves, for example, bare their teeth when threatened or ready to bite. Darwin believed that when modern man raises his upper lip in rage, it is a throwback to his ancestors' more primitive emotion, which was akin to that of the wolf.

More recently, the biologist Edward O. Wilson has added to the debate about man's emotions with some of the ideas in his 1975 book, *Sociobiology*. He argues that our value systems are influenced by the emotional responses directed from the limbic system, the brain's emotion center (see Chapter 8 for a further discussion), rather than arrived at through rational or moral choice. In this view, the limbic system acts

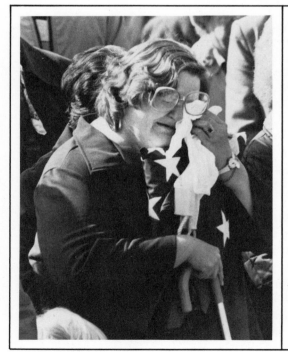

The mother of a soldier who died in Vietnam expresses her grief after being presented with an American flag at a memorial service for veterans killed in action.

as a repository of the human race's ancient emotional impulses, which are prelogical or unreasonable because they are expressed through the part of the brain we have in common with reptiles and early mammals. Thus, human nature is constrained in part by biology, including the limits to which we can reason.

What troubles many thinkers about the sociobiological view is that it accepts all that is "wrong" in human nature — racism, aggression, male dominance — by explaining those failings as part of our biological heritage. Nor does it fully explain exactly what role our moral or rational faculties *do* play in our social life.

The distinction between the brain and the mind brings up many questions. Are they *processes*, or are they *things*? Is one dependent on the other — are both dependent on each other? The biologist Sir Julian Huxley has written: "The brain alone is not responsible for mind, even though it is a necessary organ for its manifestation. Indeed, an isolated brain is a piece of biological nonsense as meaningless as an isolated individual."

A substantial body of research has been compiled to support that view, and there is general agreement on a number of key points.

Emotions involve physiological changes, along with cognitions, or thoughts. Though not always, emotions can also be accompanied by an urge to respond during or after the emotional experience. Additionally, emotions are usually triggered quickly and last only a short period of time, thus distinguishing them from moods, which tend to be more vague in degree and have a much longer duration.

If you are walking down the sidewalk and suddenly a large dog, frothing at the mouth and growling, races across the street toward you, your emotional response will almost assuredly be one of fear. Within your body, things will begin to happen. Your heart rate will increase, breathing will quicken, and you may begin to tremble.

Next, cognitive processes go to work. The thought might flash through your mind of an attack and of rabies. According to one theory, the cognitive process of sensing physiological change — the pounding heart and rapid breathing — can add to emotional intensity and even enable us to classify what emotion we are experiencing. In other words, we see the dog, feel the internal changes taking place, and think, "I am afraid."

Response, or adjustment to emotion-provoking events, is a form of coping. In the case of the attacking dog, there would likely be several means of coping: running the other way or preparing some sort of defense, for example. Interestingly, many psychologists believe that after cataloging an intense emotion like fear, the brain can reduce the physiological impact through what is called *opponent process*. This theory assumes that a chemical balance or equilibrium exists in the body, which is maintained by the brain. When an emotional experience occurs causing arousal of the sympathetic nervous system, the opponent process activates to neutralize the stress.

The Importance of Smiles and Frowns

Several studies have shown that some emotions appear to be universal; that is, they are experienced by people the world over regardless of cultural, religious, or geographic differences. Anger is one powerful emotion believed to be universal, along with fear, disgust, joy, surprise, and sadness.

Support for this assumption is based on studies of simple facial expressions. In one such study, psychologists visited a tribe in New Guinea that had never had contact with Western culture. The psychologists told the New Guinea tribesmen stories describing various emotions, then showed pictures depicting those emotions through facial expressions. Examples of the stories were, "You are angry and about to fight," or, "Your friend has come and you are happy."

Except for the expressions of fear and surprise, which the tribesmen tended to confuse (as did Americans who took the same test), the tribesmen were able to accurately match the pictures with the corresponding stories. Because the tribesmen could not possibly have *known* which pictures went with which stories, researchers concluded that some facial expressions — and the emotions they characterize — are innate among all people.

Other studies have compared the facial expressions of blind infants with those of normally sighted children. It was found that the blind babies, at an early age, exhibited *more*

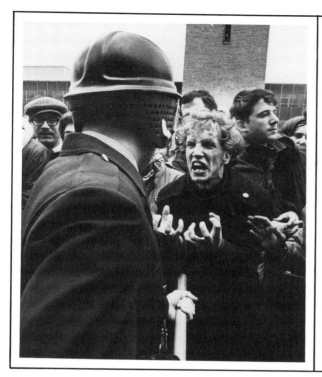

Emotions can flare up in tense, crowded settings. This student protester screams at a policeman after tear gas and riot clubs were used to break up a 1967 antiwar demonstration.

kinds of facial expressions than sighted babies of the same age. Their expressions corresponded to the appropriate emotions, too. Within a few years, though, as sighted children learned more from their environment, their repertoire of facial expressions grew larger. This fact may be explained, perhaps, by the theory that a lot of the emotions we display are merely variations on a few primary themes (love, fear, rage), and that these variations are culturally determined in some cases. The fundamental point of the studies of blind babies could be that the primary emotions are fully developed in their *mind*, directing them to use facial muscles in patterns they could never have witnessed.

Anxiety . . .

One of the most powerful emotions is anxiety. Similar to stress and fear, these three feeling states are often indistinguishable. Anxiety is caused by tension or distress, or by some vaguely anticipated tension or distress. It can be *acute*, meaning immediate, or *chronic*, meaning it can persist for long periods of time.

Anxiety occurs physiologically as a complex reaction between the brain and central nervous system. This reaction can be manifested both internally and externally by any number of common symptoms, including tightness in the stomach and muscles, sweating, dilation of the pupils, elevated blood pressure, trembling, or shaking.

Everyone experiences anxiety in the course of normal living, even small children. Some people are struck with stage fright prior to public speaking, while others are anxious about test taking. Many people experience anxiety in social situations where they must meet and interact with new people. Everyone knows the physiological feelings associated with stress: the pounding heart, flushed face, dry mouth, knots in the stomach.

Whereas some levels of anxiety can actually be positive, motivating people, say, to achieve greater goals, most stressful situations are negative and have the potential to create mild to severe mental and physical disorders. Hence, the ability to cope with stress and anxiety is crucial for mental and physical health. There are a variety of ways to cope, but unfortunately, many of them are detrimental.

. . . And Coping with It

To psychologists, coping is defined as a means to avoid, reduce, or resolve the source of stress. The most positive method for achieving this goal has been called *aggressive coping*. As the term suggests, this means taking an active part in relieving stress, either by changing our own behavior, changing the environment (the cause of the stressful situation), or by accepting the fact that sometimes a certain level of stress is unavoidable and must be adjusted to.

A coping strategy employed by Norman Cousins, when he was faced with a serious and supposedly incurable joint disease, was to foster a positive attitude. Cousins, author of the 1979 book *Anatomy of an Illness*, decided that a positive emotional outlook (and massive amounts of vitamin C) could have regenerative physical effects. In his book, he describes how he used tactics such as laughter (watching hours of slapstick comedy, for example) to improve his mood and restore his health.

There appears to be an intriguing correlation between laughter and the body's ability to ward off disease. The evidence is so strong in some people's opinion that many hospitals around the country have installed so-called laughter rooms to help sick people's moods. Saint John's Hospital and Health Center in Santa Monica, California, even has a humor channel on closed-circuit television to boost its patients' spirits.

According to an article in *Psychology Today* ("Laugh and be Well?" October 1987), some researchers believe laughter can help strengthen the body's immune system against disease. Theoretically, this is accomplished in two ways: Laughter triggers the secretion of neurotransmitters, chemicals in the brain that either block the production of immune suppressors (which put the body at greater risk of infection) or increase the production of immune enhancers (which defend the body against disease). Although this field of research, called *psychoneuroimmunology*, is still in its infancy, it is common knowledge that a hearty laugh feels good and causes the body to relax, thereby relieving stress.

Inevitably, people react to stressful conditions in negative or potentially maladaptive ways. Procrastination is a classic example of a negative coping strategy. Rather than address a problem, the procrastinator will simply put it off until later. Everyone, at one time or another, has procrastinated. It is only when negative coping becomes excessive that serious ramifications can occur.

Failure to Cope

If negative coping strategies — what Freud called defense mechanisms — are relied upon too heavily, they can lead to abnormal behavior and emotional disorders. Unable to cope with the reality of life, many people turn to drugs as a means of escape. While this strategy often relieves stress temporarily, eventually it can produce a far more serious problem. Thus, the coping strategy of drug use to reduce stress does not resolve the initial problem but merely compounds it.

Often, our attempts to cope are not made on a conscious level. Few alcoholics, in the initial stage of the disease, will even admit they have a drinking problem. Many of these negative coping strategies, according to Freudian theory, are utilized without the individual's being aware of them.

Other common defense mechanisms defined by Freud include:

• Rationalization: "It doesn't matter if I flunked the chemistry exam, I don't want to be a chemist anyway."

• Projection: The individual projects his or her anxiety onto another person. The problem drinker might say of the fellow sitting at the opposite end of the bar, "Boy, *that* guy drinks like a fish!"

• Identification: People take on the traits and characteristics of a feared or admired person or group. A student anxious about a perceived lack of intelligence might adopt the mannerisms and speech patterns of his favorite teacher to make himself feel smarter.

• Repression: For some people, stress and anxiety are so agonizing that the conscious mind, in an effort to ease its burden, simply buries thoughts and feelings in the unconscious.

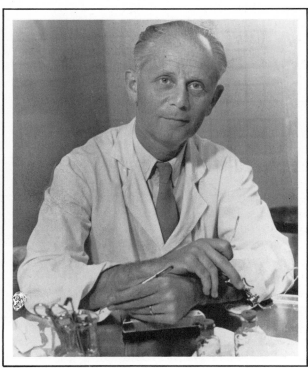

Through his experiments with white rats, the researcher Hans Selye discovered that stress causes a pattern of response — alarm, then resistance, and finally exhaustion — that he believed was also true of humans.

Freud theorized that many sexual impulses are repressed during childhood, which he believed causes emotional problems later in life.

Stress and Physical Health

Inadequate coping can cause not only emotional problems but physical illness as well. Psychologists Thomas Holmes and Richard Rahe, who devised a system to measure human anxiety levels based on common life stresses, found that individuals who show high levels of anxiety frequently show an increase in physical illness: Their tests seem to support speculation that emotional stress and anxiety are the root cause for many (some think *all*) diseases, including such common maladies as high blood pressure, and even cancer.

Researcher Hans Selye showed the harmful impact of stress in laboratory experiments with rats. Regularly injecting the rats with a substantial but nonlethal amount of poison, Selye was able to study how the animals adapted to prolonged stress. In the initial alarm period, the rats were able to marshal their defenses through the sympathetic nervous system by increasing production of adrenalin and blood sugar and by elevating heart rate to energize the body. Then, a period of recovery or resistance occurred. It seemed that the rats had returned to normal metabolic functioning. But it soon became evident that their bodies were still producing unusually high amounts of glucose and hormones to fight the poison. In the end, the prolonged stress caused an equally prolonged consumption of energy, which, in turn, led to exhaustion and ultimately death.

Selye called this sequence of events — alarm, resistance, exhaustion — the *general adaptation syndrome*, and he believed, along with other researchers, that the human nervous system responds to stressful experiences along a similar pattern.

Adolescence: Transition Time

Anxiety and stress can seem particularly intense during adolescence, a transitional period of life that presents unique emotional challenges. A time of often dramatic biological and personality changes, adolescence can be both rewarding and

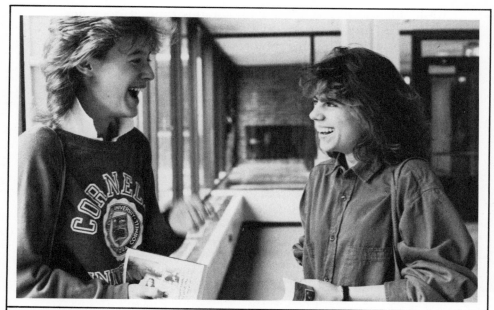

Although young adulthood can be tumultuous, many people say that some of the happiest times of their lives occurred during that period, as they experienced independence for the first time.

confounding. Many young people look forward to independence from parents and yet are apprehensive about being on their own. Adolescents must grapple with establishing a sexual identity, and they must also make important choices for education and career. The future holds great excitement, but the uncertainty of the future, and the present, can also pave the way for emotional upheavals.

In one study, 30-year-olds were asked which period of their lives had been the most difficult and confusing. The answer given by many was adolescence. The reasons? Pressure from parents and peers, to do well academically and to form successful relationships with both sexes, and the stress associated with trying to assert one's independence while still financially dependent on parents.

As in other instances, however, the range of "normal" responses to the challenges of adolescence varies widely. Many young people have rewarding experiences during adolescence, both with friends and family members. Moreover, while adolescence is often a tumultuous time, it does not necessarily have to be. Developmental psychologist Anne C. Petersen, writing on this subject in *Psychology Today*, said, "My research and that of many others suggests that although the early teen years can be quite a challenge for normal youngsters and their families, they're usually not half as bad as they are reputed to be."

Whether in the throes of adolescence or adulthood, it would seem that the ability to live a healthy emotional life has a great deal to do with understanding the nature of emotions — both from a physical and cognitive aspect — and employing positive coping strategies to deal with the inevitable stresses encountered in daily living. It is also important to realize that even extreme emotional reactions are in most cases normal responses to major stresses.

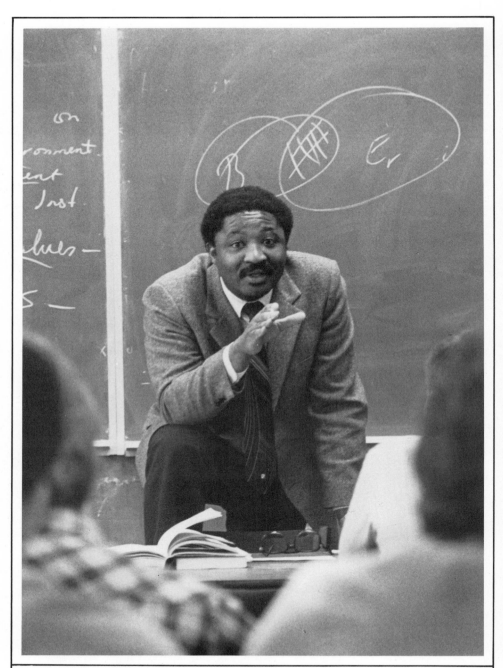

A teacher addresses his high school class. The ability to learn is a remarkable resource. Every normally functioning person is capable of learning millions of things in his or her lifetime.

CHAPTER 4

LEARNING

Man's ability to learn is far and away his most formidable resource. Without this ability, it is doubtful the human race would have survived for very long, let alone have achieved such a measure of sophistication.

What is learning, exactly? Naturally, so complex a concept has many definitions, but most psychologists accept the idea that learning consists of any relatively lasting change in behavior caused by experience.

Every normally functioning person, no matter what his or her circumstance, learns thousands, perhaps millions of lessons in the course of a lifetime. We are not born, for example, with even the most basic knowledge — that a hot stove can burn, a speeding car can maim, or that birds can fly but man cannot. Man is not alone in possessing this learning capacity, but he possesses it to a degree so much greater than other animals that his behavior has been largely freed from the forces of instinct.

Unlike man, many animals are bound by the genetics of their species, each carrying a specific genetic blueprint that predetermines behavior. Salmon swim upstream to spawn because that is their genetic destiny. Some species of bear hibernate in the winter for the same reason. These are purely instinctive behaviors, meaning they are biologically inherited, not learned.

For much of this century, the study of learning focused exclusively on behavior. Psychologists studied only the external, observable aspects of learning, largely ignoring internal mental processes. Today, however, many researchers have also come to recognize the cognitive aspects of learning. Social learning theories, as they are called, suggest that both the environment and cognitive processes play an important role in shaping learned behavior, and that through selective sorting and interpreting of information people can exert a far greater degree of control over their learning destiny than was once presumed by behaviorists.

The Conditioned Response

It is not difficult to understand why behavioral theories were predominant for so long. There are several powerful ways in which learning is affected by behavioral conditioning, and they are easily observed—and created—in the laboratory.

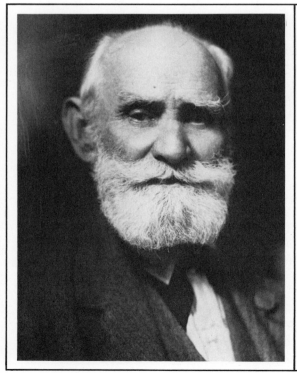

The Russian physiologist Ivan Pavlov invented a behavioral learning technique called classical conditioning by training dogs to salivate at the sound of a bell.

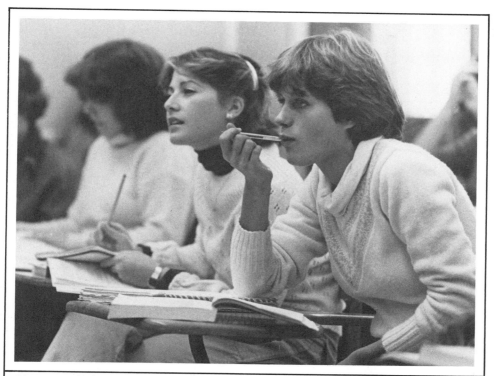

Most psychologists agree that learning consists of any lasting change in behavior that is caused by experience and that humans possess a greater capability for learning than any other animal.

Perhaps the most fundamental type of behavioral learning, discovered by the Russian physiologist Ivan Pavlov (1849–1936), is called *classical conditioning*. Experimenting with dogs, Pavlov discovered that reflex actions like salivation could be conditioned. Whenever food was placed in a dog's bowl, the dog salivated. But by introducing a neutral stimulus — a bell — just before the food was placed in the bowl, the dog soon began to salivate at the sound of the bell, before the food appeared. The animal was demonstrating a reflexive response to a previously neutral stimulus: The dog had been classically conditioned.

This may not seem a terribly important discovery until viewed in the context of human behavior. Consider, for example, the young man who is afraid of needles but nevertheless must have a shot every week as treatment for allergies. The nurse who administers the weekly shot wears a distinctive perfume. Although she tries to console the young man, prior to each injection he becomes very fearful and begins to tremble. Several weeks into the treatment, the young man is shopping at the local mall when a woman walks by wearing the same perfume as the nurse. Suddenly, for no apparent reason, the young man becomes afraid and begins to tremble.

Unwittingly, the young man has been classically conditioned. Because the nurse's perfume (the *conditioned stimulus*) has been closely associated with the fear of the needle (*the unconditioned stimulus*), when the young man smells the perfume on a different person he exhibits the same conditioned response of fear. Pavlov also discovered that a conditioned stimulus can become *generalized*, meaning a response learned in one situation may be exhibited in other, similar situations.

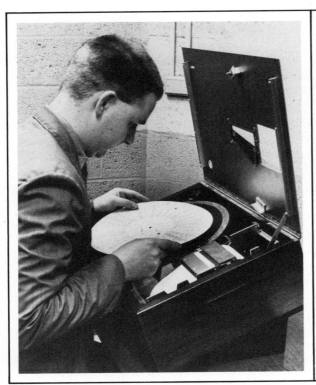

A student examines a scientific "slot machine" designed to make learning more interesting. This instrument, invented by B. F. Skinner, poses questions to students repeatedly until they have correctly answered each a satisfactory number of times.

The young man fearful of needles might begin to generalize the nurse's distinctive perfume with similar fragrances, so that eventually, many different perfumes might elicit the conditioned response of fear.

Generalization is also important because it helps people adapt to a number of similar but different situations. If you have learned that a steak knife can cut your finger, for example, the process of generalization allows you to infer that a pocket-knife or a sword could also cause the same type of injury.

Although classically conditioned learning can persist a long time, Pavlov found that if the conditioned stimulus is removed, gradually the conditioned response will disappear. This phenomenon is called *extinction*. To use the above-mentioned example, if the doctor's nurse decided to stop wearing perfume for some reason, the young man's conditioned response would eventually be extinguished and he would no longer fear the smell of the perfume.

The Case of Albert

Pavlov's research was met with great enthusiasm when it was introduced in America in the 1920s. In fact, John Watson, the American psychologist credited with founding the behaviorist school, believed that all learning could be attributed to the principles of classical conditioning.

To illustrate that point, Watson undertook the conditioning of an 11-month-old baby named Albert, who was made to fear a furry white rat. Although at first Albert had no fear of the rat, Watson paired the rat's appearance with a loud and frightening noise. Before long, Albert had been conditioned to fear the rat even when the loud noise was absent. Later, his fear was generalized to other white, furry objects, and after about one month, Albert was also afraid of a rabbit, a dog, and even a fur coat.

Such experiments with humans are not condoned today, but the story of Albert and the white rat illustrates the remarkable degree to which human behavior can be shaped. It also sheds some light on how unreasonable fears, or *phobias*, are acquired.

The claustrophobic, who fears closed-in places, understands that being terrified of elevators and telephone booths is irrational, yet the fear persists. Although the person has no idea how the claustrophobia originated, many researchers believe such phobic reactions begin as nothing more than classical conditioning: The fear was learned as a result of some conditioned response, perhaps a trauma from early childhood, and for some reason the fearful response was never extinguished.

Operant Conditioning

Another powerful type of conditioned behavior is operant, or instrumental conditioning. Popularized by B. F. Skinner, this method of learning is based primarily on learned consequences.

Unlike classical conditioning, which involves reflex action, *operant conditioning* works on a voluntary basis and is not associated with an obvious stimulus like Pavlov's bell or the nurse's perfume.

The basic tenet of operant conditioning is simple: We choose a certain behavior because we are either rewarded or punished as a consequence of it. The person who eats snails for the first time and loves them will likely eat them again. The person who eats snails for the first time and develops an upset stomach will likely avoid them in the future. This is known as the *law of effect*: Those behaviors that result in pleasant experiences will likely be repeated. Conversely, those behaviors followed by unpleasant experiences will likely be avoided.

Operant theory defines pleasant experiences as rewards, or *positive reinforcement*. Unpleasant experiences are called punishment, or *negative reinforcement*.

Skinner has dramatically shown the power of operant conditioning by teaching animals to perform complex behaviors. In a device now called a "Skinner box," for example, pigeons were conditioned to play Ping-Pong. Using positive reinforcement (rewards of food) when the birds stumbled onto correct behavior, and negative reinforcement (no food) for wrong behavior, Skinner was able to gradually shape the pigeons' behavior, bit by bit, to the desired overall task of holding paddles in their beaks and knocking a ball back and forth across a table.

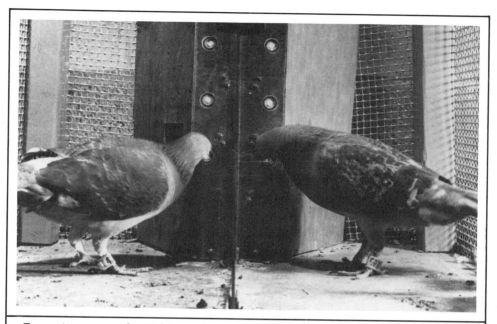

Two pigeons in the "Skinner box" designed by B. F. Skinner. In a dramatic experiment using positive and negative reinforcement, Skinner was able to train these birds to play Ping-Pong.

Sometimes the reinforcement process is not so calculated. When a reinforcer happens to follow a behavior *coincidentally*, a person may wrongly assume that the reinforcement was a consequence of the particular behavior. This is often how superstitious behavior occurs. A tennis player wears a new pair of socks and wins a key match. Subsequently, he wears the socks every time he plays, superstitiously (and wrongly) believing they are responsible for his excellent play.

All human beings are affected by the principles of operant conditioning. Moreover, we all use operant techniques in everyday life. If a friend is talking while you are trying to study, you might ignore him, thereby sending the message that you are busy. Technically, you are using negative reinforcement to shape your friend's behavior. Eventually, if you do not reward his behavior by responding, he will most likely get the picture and leave you alone.

Aversive Conditioning

When behavior is conditioned solely by negative reinforcement or punishment, it is called *aversive conditioning.* Sometimes this phenomenon occurs naturally. If you go out of doors in the winter wearing shorts and a T-shirt, the extreme cold is the negative reinforcer that will send you quickly back inside for long pants and a coat. You have been conditioned by the weather to wear proper garments.

Aversive conditioning is also used deliberately to shape behavior. Spanking children as a disciplinary measure is aversive conditioning. Denial of a positive reinforcer is also considered aversive conditioning, as when parents "ground" a teenager because of some undesired behavior.

Although aversive conditioning can be extremely effective, it is widely believed today that punishment as a learning tool is best used in conjunction with positive reinforcement. Undesirable behavior is punished (or sometimes simply ignored) while desired behavior is rewarded and praised.

Cognitive Theories of Learning

Social learning theories have taken the behaviorist approach and added a key component: cognition. According to social learning theories, learning is not only a matter of being conditioned by factors in the environment, but also a matter of mental process. The cognitive approach assumes that human beings have the capacity to select, organize, and interpret information from the environment to help choose appropriate behavior.

Social learning theorists point to the *anticipation* of reinforcement as a key motivator in behavior. This, of course, implies a cognitive factor. A particular course of action may not involve immediate reinforcement, but the anticipation of positive reinforcement in the future is inducement enough to continue the behavior. Thus a struggling actor might suffer for years taking small parts and working odd jobs in the hopes of one day getting a chance to perform on Broadway and become a star.

Another cognitive factor is *observational learning*, in which people use models — perhaps an individual or group — to observe and learn from. The young basketball enthusiast, for example, might watch professional games on television and then try to emulate what he has seen.

Although the cognitive theory of learning is far more difficult to study and measure than classical or operant conditioning, there are few psychologists today who do not acknowledge the importance of cognition in the learning process.

The Motivation Factor

There are a number of variables that influence learning. Memory is one important factor that will be discussed in the next chapter. Motivation is also crucial to the learning process.

Let's say a rat is being conditioned to run a complex maze. His reward, at the end of the maze, is food. His performance is based on learned responses, but also on motivation. If the rat is hungry he is motivated to run the maze quickly. If he has just eaten and is satiated, he is not motivated and therefore runs the maze slowly.

As defined by psychologists, motivation is a feeling state brought on by a *need* that prompts behavior. The behavior is usually directed at fulfilling the need. When we feel thirsty, we are motivated to get something to drink.

There are many kinds of motives. Primary motives are biological in nature — the need for food and water, shelter and safety. Other motives appear to have no biological necessity but are nevertheless important.

As we saw in earlier chapters, Freud believed human beings have unconscious motives that are sexual and aggressive in nature and are responsible for many types of behavior. There is also the motivation of achievement, which drives people to excel, say, in sports or academics or their chosen career. The young person who is highly motivated toward achievement as a doctor will probably pay much greater attention in chemistry class than another person who is motivated to be a musician and has no interest in chemistry. Motives play a crucial role in an individual's capacity to learn.

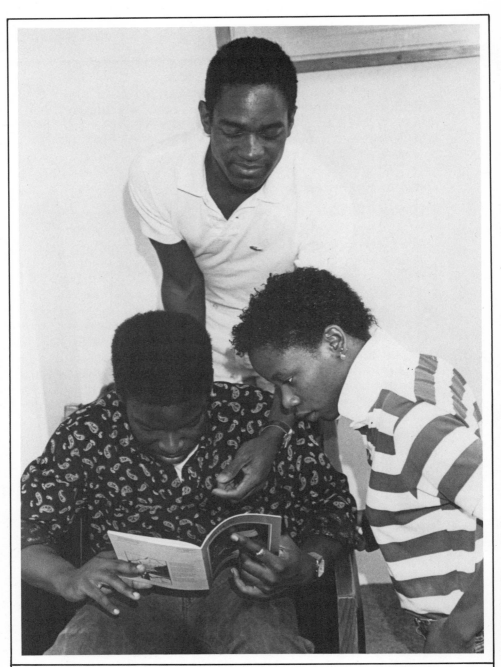

Youths work on their schoolwork. Each new thought sets off a series of electrical impulses and chemical messages in the brain, which in turn translates the thought into a memory to be stored.

CHAPTER 5

MEMORY

A friend who moved away years ago comes back to the old neighborhood for a visit. Although you have not seen or really thought about the person for many years, upon meeting him again you immediately remember his name and that he played the trumpet.

Similarly, without effort you can also remember the telephone numbers of several friends, multiplication tables, the smell of turpentine, and you can recall as many as 40,000 words and the grammatical structure of at least one highly complex language, English. And, of course, sometimes you can't remember the year your mother was born.

Such are the riddles of memory, the tremendous faculty by which human beings process, store, and retrieve a multitude of facts and a wide array of information.

The Amazing Brain

With recent advances in technology, scientists studying the human brain have gained a much greater knowledge of how its electrical and chemical processes affect a variety of important bodily functions, including memory.

To understand the nature of memory — how and why we store, remember, and forget perceptions — we must first understand the basic operation of the brain, the body's most complicated organ. Gene Bylinsky, a science writer, elegantly describes the workings of the human brain this way:

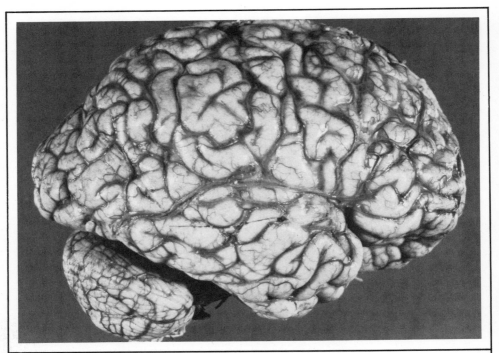

A normal human brain. Some researchers believe that neurotransmitters, the chemical messengers in the brain, relay information from neuron to neuron and may be the key to memory.

Under an electron microscope, the brain looks like a tropical rain forest. Neurons resembling clumps of uprooted trees intermingle with thick vinelike axons, through which the neurons transmit electrical signals, to form a seemingly chaotic, jungle-like growth. Like a rain forest, the brain is a noisy place; the neurons fire electrical pulses constantly. It's also wet, drenched with chemicals. And like a forest, it's living, constantly changing. For example, dendrites, the rootlike receivers for electrical impulses sent to the neurons, can grow new protrusions in minutes in response to new experiences. Sheets of glial cells sweep through the brain like squalls, apparently to nourish the sprouting neurons.

A new impression — a sight, a thought, a sound, even a smell — generates electrical pulses that race through the neurons and their connecting networks of dendrites and axons.

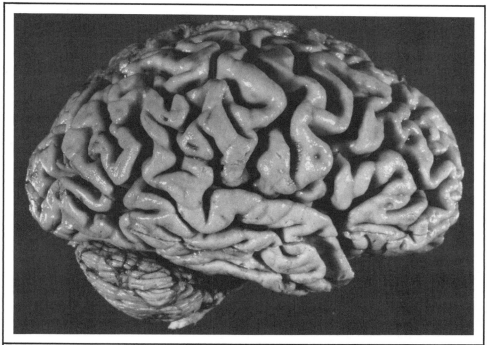

The deepened cavities between the folds of this brain, which is afflicted with Alzheimer's disease, indicate degeneration. Alzheimer's is a disease that seriously impairs memory.

Where neurons meet lie narrow slits known as synapses. The electrical signal never crosses a synapse. Instead, it causes the release of a chemical signal substance called a neurotransmitter.

Neurotransmitters may be the key to remembering. Each one of the brain's neurotransmitter molecules is a vital link in the chain of memory, relaying information from one neuron to another in as short a time span as .5 milliseconds. No one is sure exactly how many different neurotransmitters there are, but research is under way to discover as yet unknown neurotransmitters and identify their exact roles. It is believed that some of these chemical substances are responsible for highly specialized or even unique activities within the brain.

People suffering from Alzheimer's disease, an incurable deteriorative disorder that seriously impairs memory, are often found to have a shortage of the neurotransmitter acetylcholine. In some cases, patients whose acetylcholine levels were increased by the use of drugs have shown some revival of memory capacity. At the other end of the age scale, children who are malnourished have been found to suffer from reduced learning and memory-formation ability. A child's social environment may play a role, but the insufficient organic makeup in the brain that can result from malnourishment is an undeniable cause as well.

Memories are represented in the brain through a series of electrical impulses and chemical messages. Although this may well account for how information is recorded, stored, and retrieved, there are many other mental operations to consider concerning the nature of memory.

Levels of Memory

Why, for example, can we vividly remember an event from early childhood, but forget an event that happened only days ago? The answer is that there is more than one kind of memory. In fact, psychologists distinguish among three basic types of memory: sensory, short-term, and long-term.

Sensory memory, the most limited of human memories (though only in terms of how long it remains stored as information), applies to those extremely fleeting memories derived from the senses: a glimpse of a falling leaf, a faint noise in the distance, the feel of a cool breeze on the back of the neck. Every person has thousands of sensory memories during the course of a day, and although these memories quickly decay, almost as soon as they register in the brain, if they are attended to and interpreted, they can be easily processed and transferred to another type of memory, short-term memory.

As its name suggests, short-term memory does not mean deep-seated knowledge, but it is far more lasting than sensory memory. Moreover, short-term memory is often thought of as a kind of memory clearinghouse, a repository of pertinent information to be processed into long-term memory, or of less resilient information that will be deemed unnecessary and discarded.

A typical example of short-term memory: You become lost while driving. A passerby gives you brief but detailed directions, which you listen to, repeat aloud, and remember until you can jot them down a minute or so later.

The reason you remembered the directions long enough to write them down is that they were temporarily stored in short-term memory. Tests have shown that unless short-term material is rehearsed, that is, repeated verbally or mentally, or transferred to long-term memory, it will be remembered for only about 15 or 20 seconds.

The lifespan on information in the long-term memory is much more variable. Material may be stored for as little as an hour or as long as a lifetime. There is virtually no limit to the amount of information that can be stored in long-term memory (the amount may have *practical* limits for most people, however), and the material can range from a complicated physics equation to the ability to recognize yourself in the mirror. As you might expect, long-term memories take longer to form in the mind, because a longer neuronal chain must be built to store them.

Most long-term memories are never called upon actively, but their dormancy does not seem to matter. Especially in elderly persons, memories from the distant past, as far back as 70 or 80 years, can be triggered and revived with complete

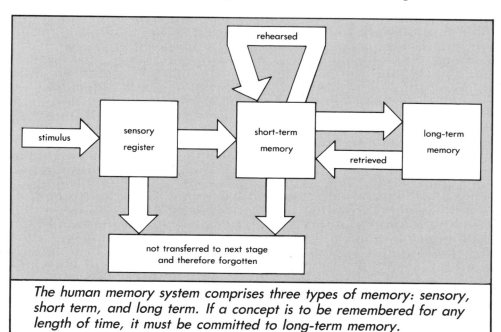

The human memory system comprises three types of memory: sensory, short term, and long term. If a concept is to be remembered for any length of time, it must be committed to long-term memory.

clarity. One reason some of the elderly "live in the past" is that as all of their memories fade, long-term memory, being the largest storehouse, begins to represent a larger overall portion of what they can recall. What is most amazing about remembering a face or name from the very distant past is not that someone can do it, but that the initial perception through chemical neurotransmission may have lasted as little as an hour.

How We Remember

The process by which information is stored in the brain, for all categories of memory, is called *encoding*. We encode music, for example, by translating the notes we hear into electrical impulses in the brain, which are then stored, and later retrieved, via neurotransmitters.

Most encoding is thought to be organized, or networked, by concepts. We form concepts as a foundation of knowledge, then mentally file new information according to the appropriate concept. In this fashion specific networks of information are created.

Suppose, for example, someone asks you to name the third president of the United States. To arrive at the answer, you need not sort through information, say, on oceans of the world or the history of Rome. The concept of presidents somehow triggers the retrieval of the appropriate network of information while avoiding other extraneous networks. When you retrieve from your long-term memory that the answer is Thomas Jefferson, you will have drawn on grade-school knowledge, and will probably be able to draw on that memory at any time during your life.

Retrieving stored information is generally thought to be similar in nature to the encoding process, in that the information is remembered according to specific concepts and networks. There appears to be support for this theory from studies done with stroke patients who suffered memory impairment. (A stroke is a rupture or obstruction of an artery of the brain, often causing paralysis or permanent disability.) In one study, stroke victims with memory loss had forgotten only the names of fruits and vegetables, but nothing else.

Association and retrieval cues are an integral component of the concept/network model of memory. A new piece of

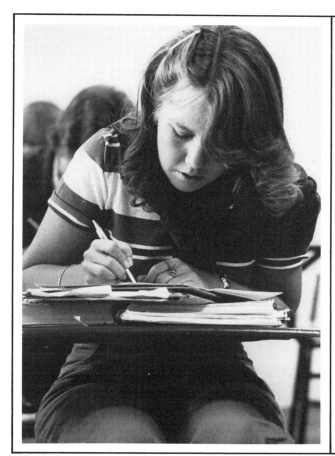

information to be stored is often paired with another piece of information already in storage. You might associate the numbers of a lock combination, 1–22–48, with your mother's birthday, January 22, 1948.

Similarly, retrieval cues are bits of information that help us remember other information. Say that someone asks you who invented the telephone. You are sure you know the answer but you just cannot come up with the name (this common feeling is known as the "tip of the tongue" phenomenon). Using a retrieval cue, you recall that the phone company is known as the Bell System, which then brings to mind the name Alexander Graham Bell, the inventor. Often a whole series of retrieval clues may be needed to recollect a certain fact from the memory, such as the names of the six Central American nations.

Information may also be associated visually, using mental images. A striking illustration of this was the case of the Russian man known as "S.", whose capacity to remember was limitless. During regular testing over a 30-year period, psychologists were astounded by the man's perfect recall. S. could listen to or look at lengthy strings of numbers or words and recall them weeks, months, even 15 years later.

How did he do it? S. said that he changed the words or numbers, or whatever the material happened to be, into vivid and consistent images that he could see in his mind, and in some cases, could taste and smell. His image for the number 2, for example, was a high-spirited woman. Unfortunately, his spectacular powers of recall became a terrible hindrance, for he was unable to stop the image process. Simple activities like reading a newspaper or talking to someone would conjure countless vivid images in his brain. Ultimately, S. was unable to grasp complicated ideas or concentrate on one thing for any length of time.

Strategies for Remembering

For most people, imagery, association, and networking are vital in both the learning and memory processes. Although these workings are often utilized automatically, they can also be practiced in a more deliberate way to enhance memory. A simple memory strategy universally used by students as well as adults is repetition. Reading a class assignment not once but many times will help prepare the material for easier future retrieval.

A series of words can often be converted into a memory-aiding system called a *mnemonic device* (pronounced ne-MAH-nic). The principle of a mnemonic device is to help the mind reproduce an unfamiliar idea, or several dissociated ideas, by connecting them with some artificial whole. Rhymes are one effective and common strategy for doing this — a simple one is "*i* before *e* except after *c*." The rhymes can be somewhat more elaborate, too, such as the one for remembering which months do not have 31 days:

Thirty days hath September,
April, June, and November.

Acronyms are another common form of mnemonic device, in which the first letters of a series of words are stitched together to form a word of their own. *Scuba*, for instance, stands for self-contained underwater breathing apparatus. The fact that hundreds of such acronyms are part of our common parlance is a testament to the usefulness of retrieval cues as a system to aid memory.

Mnemonics can also be complex visual images. The Russian S. often memorized strings of words by visualizing a familiar street. As he mentally walked down the street, he would place each word, in sequence, in a particular and familiar spot. To retrieve the information, he would simply take that mental walk again, stopping at each familiar place to pick up the word he had placed there.

Studies have shown that people who use strategies like mnemonics can indeed increase their capacity to learn and recall information. Still, no matter what strategies are employed, people do forget.

Theories of Forgetting

A number of psychologists suggest that some forgetting is actually a good thing. If people were able to remember everything, as did S., their minds would be a constant jumble and they would not be able to function well at all.

A major part of forgetting, some theorists believe, is improper encoding. If information is not encoded correctly at the outset, it will naturally be difficult to retrieve. For example, if you are watching the evening news on television while talking to a friend, you might not remember exactly what the anchorwoman just said, although you heard something about congressional hearings. If someone later asks you what happened at the congressional hearings that day, you will not be able to retrieve the information because it was never properly stored in the first place.

Another factor in forgetting is called *interference*. If you cannot recall what color the family car was 10 years ago, it might be that other stored information — including the color of the family cars since then — is interfering with that initial memory.

In years past, one of the most widely held assumptions about forgetting — known as the *decay theory* — presumed that if you fail to use information in long-term memory, eventually it can decay and disappear. This notion has been chal-

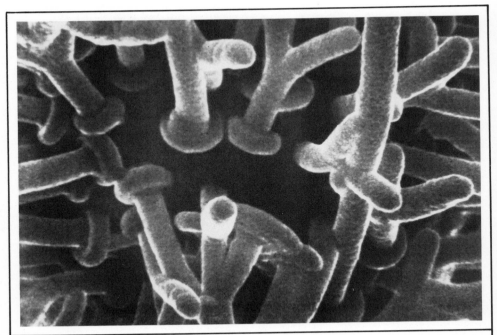

A magnified photograph of the synaptic knobs. Some researchers believe that information must travel across these synaptic connections twice in order to be retained in long-term memory.

lenged, however. Recent studies of neurotransmitters in the brain suggest that old memories do not have to decay to make room for new memories. Furthermore, some stroke victims with brain damage found themselves remembering previously "forgotten" information. In one case, a stroke victim began to speak a language he had not heard, read, or spoken in years.

Emotions, Memory, and Forgetting

The link between emotions and memory capacity is undeniable, though it is a difficult one to quantify. Family quarrels, for instance, can dominate a person's thoughts long after the event, because each time the fight is retold or rethought the perceptions of it are encoded again. It is then likely to stay in long-term memory, colored somewhat by either the less objective or more objective interpretations given it after the fact. On the more everyday level, anything we feel strongly about — whatever we have some emotional or personal attachment to, such as a person, place, song, book, or adventure — is much more likely to stay in the memory. This causal link between a deep feeling and its memory, however, is not guaranteed.

There is also the theory of motivated forgetting, which proposes that people sometimes seek to purposely forget. *Repression*, the Freudian term for burying painful feelings, is an emotional reaction to an event that the holder is motivated to forget. A conscious or an unconscious effort can be made to forget the details or the entirety of a lovers' quarrel, if it causes too much emotional damage.

As further research is done on neurotransmission, on memory decay in the elderly or the injured, and on the emotionally determined components of memory, we will have a clearer idea of human limits and capacities. But given the enormous complexity of the brain and its ever-changing chemistry in every individual, theories about memory may have to remain as general or as partial as they were in the past.

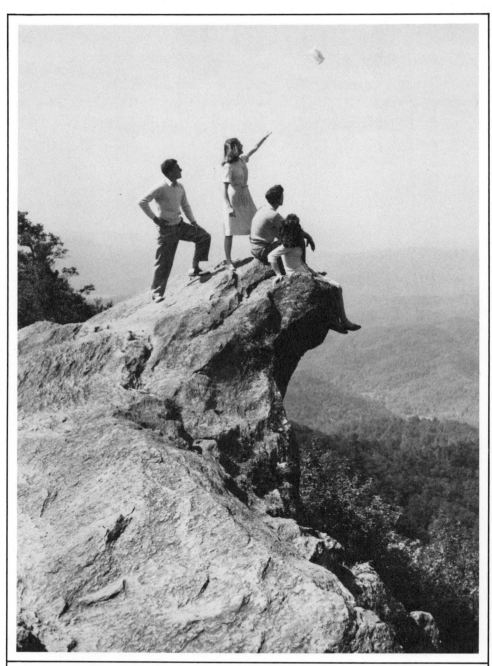

Humans often take for granted their ability to sense and perceive their environment. But new situations, such as unfamiliar surroundings, can heighten these perceptions.

CHAPTER 6

SENSATION AND PERCEPTION

Human beings are so finely tuned to their surroundings that the remarkable ability to sense and perceive those surroundings is largely taken for granted. We walk down a tree-lined path on a crisp autumn day and experience a whole spectrum of sensory events: many-colored leaves falling to the ground, the steam from our own breath, the crackle of acorns underfoot, the warmth of the sun on our cheeks.

But without the senses — vision, hearing, smell, taste, and touch — we would have no way of knowing what a tree looks like or how the sun feels. In fact, we would not be able to experience or collect any information from the environment. Simply put, our senses connect us to the world.

Sensory organs like the eyes, ears, nose, and mouth are extremely sensitive and specialized receptors that gather information from the environment and send it along for processing to the brain and nervous system. The act of processing and interpreting that information into thoughts, ideas, and judgments is called *perception*.

Consider the baseball player stepping into the batter's box. Sixty feet six inches away stands the pitcher, holding a ball roughly the size of an orange. Rearing back, the pitcher

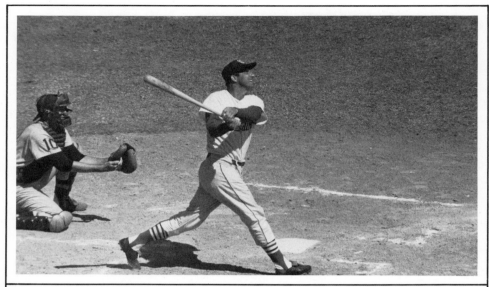

Stan Musial of the St. Louis Cardinals at bat in 1961. Although hitting a ball may appear to be a simple task, it is actually a complex combination of sensory and perceptual actions.

takes aim and lets the ball fly toward home plate at better than 90 miles an hour. In an instant, the batter sees the ball coming and tightens his grip on the bat.

In that extremely brief moment a vast amount of sensory and perceptual activity takes place. Responding to electro-magnetic energy — rays of light — reflecting from the pitcher and the ball, the batter's eyes gather a range of information and immediately convert it into the electrochemical signals that the brain and nervous system understand. As the ball approaches, receptors in the skin and muscles sense the phys-ical pressure of the bat. Additionally, the batter concentrates his attention exclusively on the pitcher and the ball, filtering out other sensory data such as the roar of the crowd and the other players' movements on the field.

Once the senses have completed these tasks, perception takes over. Information received from the various sensory receptors is organized and interpreted, and with incredible speed, motor action is initiated: The batter perceives the ball's speed, distance, and trajectory, and swings.

The Nature of Sensation

Any external energy, such as light or sound, is called a *stimulus*. The receptor cells that make up the various sensory organs, then, are responsible for the detection of stimuli. Once a stimulus is detected by the sensory organs, the information is converted into electrochemical signals that will be interpreted by the brain and nervous system. This conversion process is called *transduction*. A record player, for example, transduces, or converts, the information on a record album into the electrical impulses compatible with the operation of the stereo amplifier. The speakers, in turn, transduce the electronic impulses from the amplifier into mechanical energy, or sound waves. The sound waves are sensed by the human ear and are further transduced, this time into electrochemical messages that travel through the brain and finally result in the *perception* of music. Because this last stage of transduction is subject to competing processes that may be occurring in the brain at the same time, not everything that is sensed is perceived. The brain is selective when it comes to perception.

The organs of sense are also very selective. Every species of animal has its own distinct set of sensory mechanisms, which can be seen as special capabilities for special needs. Bats, for example, have extremely poor vision but exceptional high-pitch hearing for nocturnal hunting and navigation. Some species of insects are deaf except for the limited range of sound frequencies made by their predators.

Human beings have extremely well-developed sensory mechanisms. Studies have shown that on a clear night the human eye is capable of seeing a candle flame more than 30 miles away. The sense of smell is so delicate one can detect the scent of a single drop of perfume in a three-bedroom apartment. And the 10,000 or so taste buds in the mouth can quickly distinguish among a broad range of foods.

Human sensory mechanisms respond to a tremendous variety of stimuli, but individually, each sensory organ, as well as individual receptors within the organs, has its own narrow range of operation. The *somatosensory* systems, commonly called the "skin senses," respond to warmth, cold, pain and pressure. Similarly, there are millions of receptor cells in the eye, and each is sensitive to a specific segment of the light spectrum.

The human ear, although capable of hearing sounds in the approximate range of 20 to 20,000 hertz (a frequency measured in cycles per second), is incapable of hearing sounds above and below that range. We cannot, for example, hear the high-pitched noise emitted by bats, or many of the sounds dogs and cats regularly discern.

Sensory messages are mixed and integrated in an area in the brain stem called the *locus coeruleus*, a small but very important part of the brain. The locus coeruleus then sends its messages to many other parts of the brain, including the limbic system, which controls emotions. It is thought that the influence of many drugs on our sensations and perceptions occurs because of the way that these drugs affect the locus coeruleus.

There is evidence that psychedelic drugs such as mescaline and LSD act to stimulate the activity of cells in the locus coeruleus. These hyperactive cells then pass on their electrochemical messages to the higher brain centers where they are translated into perception, thought, and emotion. The result is that normal sights and sounds may be given new and frightening interpretations. Thus, when the British writer Aldous Huxley took mescaline, he panicked. He later wrote that it seemed his personality was "disintegrating under a pressure of reality greater than a mind accustomed to living most of the time in a cozy world of symbols could possibly bear."

Because so many drugs affect our perception of external reality, it is important to understand how the mind turns sensations into perceptions. This is one of the more mysterious talents of the brain.

The Nature of Perception

Unlike sensory mechanisms, which operate more or less automatically based on the intensity of stimuli, perception requires interpretation and is therefore a cognitive function. In fact, perception provides the basis for all higher cognitive skills, such as memory and learning.

Perception is the process by which human beings transform sensory material into thoughts and ideas. Whereas sen-

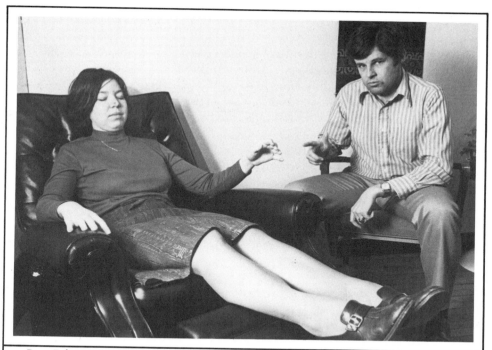

Dr. Edwin B. Fischer, a psychologist at Washington University, uses hypnotism to help patients overcome their fear of situations or objects that they perceive to be threatening.

sation connects us to the world, perception allows us to make judgments about the world. And, just as each species of animal has unique sensory mechanisms, individual humans have unique perceptual processes. These individual perceptual differences are explained by the way that sensory material is organized and interpreted in the human brain.

Consider the case of two people who speak different languages. Listening to a sentence of, say, German, one of them is baffled, while the other is able to take the same stimuli and understand it, enabling him to draw conclusions or make plans. In this case, the person who speaks German is, on the basis of learning and memory, able to *process* the verbal stimuli to a far greater degree than one who does not.

To take another case, consider two people with the same injury, a broken leg. One of them might experience agonizing pain, while the other may hardly seem bothered. In this case, instead of a difference in learning and memory, the two people may be exhibiting a difference in the chemistry of their brains or nervous systems. It has been discovered, for example, that a substance in the brain — called *endorphin* — is a natural painkiller, and may be present to varying degrees in different people, enabling some to tolerate more pain than others.

In general, however, the organization and interpretation of sensory data is less complicated than linguistic perception and more complicated than the perception of pain. Probably the most fascinating studies of perception have focused on this middle area, the perception of visual stimuli. Because it lends itself to objective measurement and statistical analysis, visual perception has revealed many basic laws of perceptual organization.

Perceiving Visual Objects

We sense many isolated stimuli every second, but we do not usually *perceive* isolated stimuli — we perceive *things*. That is, we automatically interpret our sensations in order to per-

Figure 1: Gestalt Principles of Grouping.

Proximity (dot pattern)	Proximity: The dots at left can be seen as grouped in either horizontal or vertical rows, but in the other two groups changes in the proximity of the dots causes us to automatically perceive vertical columns in the middle and horizontal rows on the right.
Similarity (rows of dots)	Similarity: The similarity of color here makes us see these dots as forming black and gray squares rather than as a row of black and gray dots.
Continuity (broken circle and square)	Closure: Even though the lines here are broken, we still see these figures as a circle and a square because we tend to close up or fill in missing parts of these shapes.
Closure (dotted crossing lines labeled A, B, C, D)	Continuity: We are much more likely to see the figures on the far left as being made up of two lines, A to B and C to D, than we are to see it as a figure made up of lines A to D and C to B, or of A to C and B to D.
Symmetry [ ] [ ] [ ] ( ) ( ) ( )	Symmetry: We are much more likely to see this as a row of six figures than as a row of twelve figures, because we tend to organize stimuli into symmetrical figures.

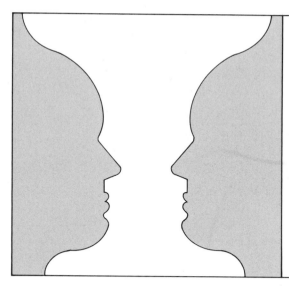

Figure 2: Gestalt Figure-Ground Organization. *People tend to perceive objects according to what they believe the background and foreground to be. For example, if the foreground in this picture is perceived to be black, the picture is of an urn. If it is perceived to be white, the picture is of two faces.*

ceive specific objects. Psychologists have arrived at several principles by which we are able to do this.

In the 1930s and 1940s a group of scientists called *Gestalt* psychologists arrived at some of the most fundamental of these principles. These included the *principles of grouping* (see figure 1), which refers to the tendency to organize isolated stimuli into groups or units on the basis of such factors as proximity (closeness), similarity, and continuity. Another Gestalt principle is called *figure-ground organization* (see figure 2); this refers to the fact that we tend to perceive things as standing out against a background, and to interpret or identify things according to what we perceive to be the background and foreground.

Still another organizing principle may be seen in the fact that while we receive a constantly changing array of sensations, we perceive many aspects of the world in an unchanging way. Thus, as you walk around your desk, your visual system will receive different patterns of stimulation with each step you take — but you will still "see" the same desk. This ability to see or discern constants in an ever-changing world of sensations is called *perceptual constancy*.

There are many more subprinciples that explain our perception of visual objects, but the general point is that perception is a far more complicated process than sensation, and

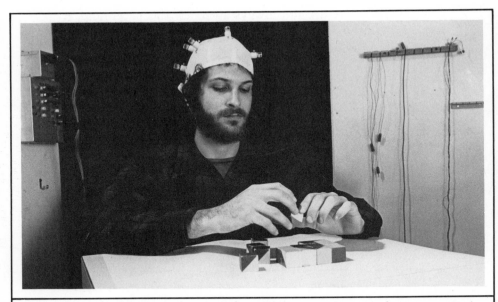

This subject is being monitored by a device that measures brain activity as he performs a perceptual excercise. Such experiments can help researchers discover how the brain recognizes patterns.

can be approached scientifically from many more perspectives. One of these — attention — is a crucial factor in learning, and provides a theoretical link between sensation and perception.

Attention: Selective Perception

As you read this, there are no doubt many other stimuli in your environment that your organs of sense are processing. If you are sitting, the pressure of your body is creating many sensations of touch; there may also be many sounds around you. This sort of phenomenon — your ability to screen out these other, competing sensations and to concentrate on what you are reading—is the focus of the study of attention.

Like many other higher processes in the brain, attention is not fully understood, but experiments suggest that at some level of processing in the brain, sensations are screened or filtered, so that only those of immediate interest or utility manage to make it through to consciousness. It is interesting, however, that we are not always aware of this screening. It has been shown, for example, that in a crowded room full of many different conversations a person can screen out almost all of the other conversations but will still notice the sound of his or her own name if it occurs in one of the screened-out conversations. In instances such as this, it seems clear that some unconscious, perhaps conditioned, response mechanism is in operation. It has also been theorized that drugs such as marijuana may erase this screening mechanism, so that *all* sensations take on equal importance in the consciousness of the user.

Because it is so important to the learning process, attention has always been the subject of great interest. Is the ability to concentrate a product of training? Or is it perhaps more physiological, and hence more dependent on general good health or even heredity? Evidence suggests that, as in so many other areas of psychology, there is no single answer. Practice and training certainly can improve concentration, but more physiological factors may also play a role.

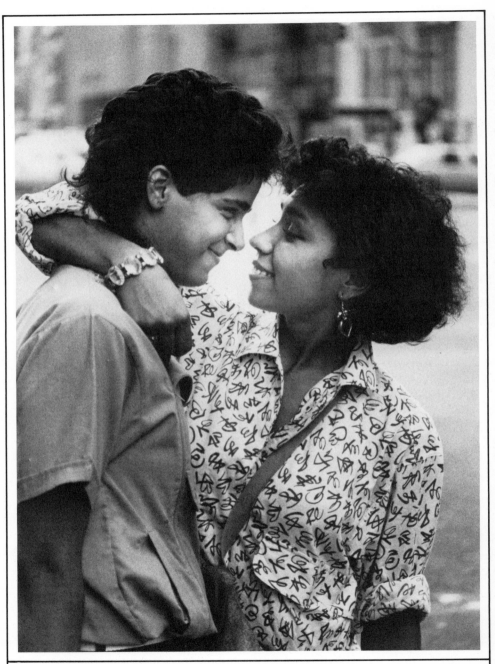

Human beings have a biological drive for sexual activity, just as we have drives for food and water. This sexual drive is more openly expressed and accepted today than in past generations.

CHAPTER 7

HUMAN SEXUALITY

American perception of sexuality has changed profoundly during the past several decades. The sexual revolution of the 1960s paved the way for a sexual freedom that today brings us everything from call-in sex-therapy shows on television to explicit lingerie advertisements. On the less frivolous side, however, once-taboo issues such as homosexuality and incest are now more openly addressed in our society.

But does being more sexually open as a culture mean we are any better equipped to understand the nature of sexuality — the psychological similarities and distinctions between men and women?

Although that question is difficult to answer with any certainty, there can be little doubt but that human beings are sexual creatures. We have a biological drive for sexual activity, just as we have drives for food and water. In fact, our sexual natures present themselves shortly after conception when gender, the sexual characteristics of maleness or femaleness, becomes apparent.

The X and Y of Gender

Gender is actually determined at conception, by information transmitted on one of the 23 chromosomes contained in the father's sperm. An X chromosome denotes female and a Y chromosome denotes male. All female eggs already contain

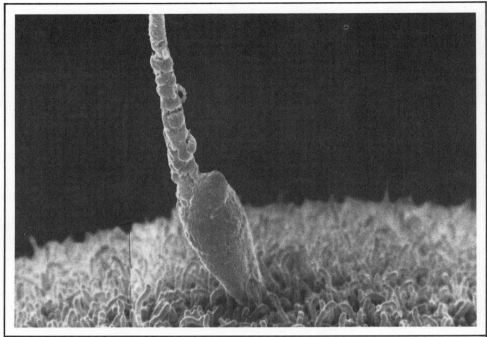

A sperm fertilizes a human egg. Gender — the maleness or femaleness of the embryo — is determined at conception.

an X, or female, chromosome, so an egg fertilized by an X chromosome will become a female (XX) while an egg fertilized by a Y chromosome will become a male (XY).

Gender becomes apparent about six weeks after conception when the gonads, which are sex glands, develop into either testes in males or ovaries in females.

Hormones produced in the gonads determine not only how the reproductive organs will develop but are also vital for their interaction with a part of the brain called the *hypothalamus*, which affects secondary sexual characteristics during puberty. Aside from regulating sexual processes, the hypothalamus helps the body maintain balance and equilibrium and also monitors such internal factors as body temperature.

Without the presence of the male hormone androgen, for example, the hypothalamus will maintain a pattern of hormone production consistent with female development. In fact, it appears that overall, males develop sexually from the female pattern. If androgens are present in the male embryo, which they normally are, the hypothalamus maintains the production pattern of those hormones so that at puberty, the male will develop secondary sexual characteristics such as facial hair and deepening of the voice.

Sexuality: A Relative Term

Although gender is clearly a genetic function, environmental influences such as societal customs dictate to a great degree how an individual's sexuality may be expressed. In some cultures, for example, homosexual relationships are permitted and even encouraged before heterosexual marriage. In other cultures, masturbation among children is permitted, as are polygamous marriages.

Not surprisingly, studies have shown that the average amount of sexual activity in our society is considered permissive by some cultures and repressive by others.

For example, on the tiny island of Inis Beag, off the coast of Ireland, the population exhibits what Americans would consider an extremely low level of sexual activity. Children are punished for exhibiting any kind of sexuality, even sexual talk. In fact, boys and girls are largely segregated. Among adults, celibacy — choosing not to marry or engage in sexual intercourse — is not unusual, and marriages are often arranged matter-of-factly, without regard for emotional attachment. Furthermore, the islanders believe that sexual intercourse itself is a debilitating act.

Gender Identity and the Nature-Nurture Issue

Individual gender roles and identities — that is, the ways men and women act and perceive themselves as masculine and feminine — are influenced both by nature (through hormones and genetic heritability) and by nurture (environmental factors such as social and religious custom). The extent to which either nature or nurture is dominant, however, is still a topic open to much debate.

Whether men and women are *emotionally* different as a function of their biology is yet another question. Although many male/female stereotypes were once accepted as factual (for instance, the view that men are naturally more aggressive and less emotional than women, and that women are more submissive and less self-reliant than men), the belief that these sorts of roles are ingrained in the species is now challenged on many fronts. In the industrialized world, and especially in America, women today are shrinking the social, economic, and political gap between themselves and men. This fact lends support to the theory that environmental factors, including learned behavior, dictate the emotional differences between the sexes.

The Nurture Argument

It is widely believed that learned, not inborn, behavior is the crucial influencing factor in sexuality. This theory suggests that individuals learn to act like males or females through a process called *sex typing*, whereby societal expectations about how men and women should act are inculcated almost from birth.

Although the gender gap is indeed narrowing in some societies, various studies have shown that in America even so-called liberated parents still tend to treat male offspring differently than female offspring. For example, fathers who play with baby girls treat them more gently than they do baby boys. When cooing to a baby, parents make different noises for girls than for boys. And mothers tend to feed boys more than girls.

Some researchers have even suggested that because children are so consistently exposed to sex typing from parents, teachers, peers, and the media, their entire cognitive styles are affected. Because of societal expectations about sexuality, they argue, children learn early on how to behave and perceive the world from either a distinctly masculine or feminine viewpoint.

The Nature Argument

Many psychologists, however, see gender as a biological imperative; they believe gender identity is genetically influenced by the production of hormones. Males produce the hormone androgen. Women produce the hormone estrogen. These psychologists theorize that these hormones program

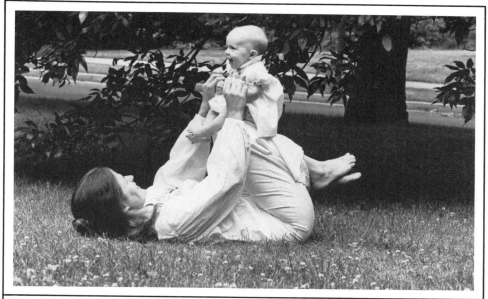

Supporters of the nurture theory believe that a person's sexual identity is established during infancy and that there are distinct differences in how male and female babies are treated.

the fetal brain to react with certain masculine or feminine tendencies.

Animal studies, for example, have shown that changing the hormonal balance of rats before or shortly after birth results in male rats showing female attributes as they mature, and female rats exhibiting male attributes. Moreover, a study of women whose mothers had been subjected to unusually high amounts of the male hormone androgen during pregnancy showed that, as a group, the women in later life were in many ways more "masculine" than "feminine." They were tomboys as children, liked to roughhouse rather than play with dolls, and preferred wearing pants to wearing dresses. As adolescents, they showed little interest in boys or baby-sitting and later expressed misgivings about marriage and motherhood.

The Phenomenon of Love

The majority of men and women in the world are hetero-sexuals who grow up to fall in love with someone of the opposite sex, marry, and raise a family. But how do people fall in love? Are there any scientific reasons for attraction and love, or is it simply a matter of chance?

Again, there is no precise answer. In fact, from a scientific standpoint there is really very little known about the feeling state of love. Some researchers believe that sexual attraction is linked in part to the olfactory senses, that is, people are attracted by various bodily odors. Other studies have shown that the most important ingredient for friendship — a vital factor for a love relationship — is not personality or similar interests but rather close proximity; we tend to make friends with people who are nearby. Furthermore, because love is such a highly subjective feeling state and involves so many different emotions, psychologists trying to study it have had a difficult task of trying to distinguish feelings of love from feelings of "like."

One theory of why love occurs is based on the phenomenon of mistaken emotions. The misattribution theory suggests that when a man or woman meets another person and is attracted, that attraction might have been confused with some other emotion the person was feeling at the time.

In one experiment illustrating misattribution, men were exposed to an attractive woman after they had just had the frightening experience of crossing an old rickety bridge over a deep gorge. As they stepped off the bridge, the attractive woman, who was helping with the experiment, asked the men to write a story about what had just happened. The stories these men wrote contained much more sexual imagery than those of another group of men who had crossed a well-built bridge that did not provoke fear.

Researchers concluded that the men on the rickety bridge were first aroused by fear and then, seeing the attractive woman, misattributed that fear for sexual arousal. If so, then the conclusion could be drawn that people may also misattribute other strong emotions as being feelings of love.

Any discussion of sexuality today must raise the topic of AIDS (Acquired Immune Deficiency Syndrome). This deadly virus, which can be transmitted through sexual activity (it is also spread through infected hypodermic needles), has reached epidemic levels in various parts of the world and is believed to be carried by perhaps a million Americans. There is as yet no cure for it.

What affect will AIDS have on modern sexuality, and hence on the emotional content of our lives? Although it may be too early to speculate, there does seem to be a trend away from sexual permissiveness. In the 1960s, proponents of the sexual revolution coined the phrase "Make love, not war." With the advent of AIDS, today's new sexual bywords seem to be "safe sex."

Sexual Deviancy

Although religious and societal customs dictate for many what is sexually appropriate and inappropriate, there are so many different religious and cultural beliefs that it hardly makes sense to label various sexual behaviors as right or wrong. There are exceptions, however, and two of those exceptions are incest and rape. Incest is defined as sexual relations between closely related persons, usually occurring between a father and daughter. Rape is sexual intercourse coerced through violence or intimidation. These forms of sexuality oppose most social norms so radically that they are labeled as sexually deviant behavior.

Homosexuality was once thought to be a form of sexual deviancy, although it is not considered so today by the American Psychiatric Association. Most psychologists define homosexuals as individuals who derive primary sexual gratification from members of the same sex. The cause of this sexual orientation has for many years been a topic of great interest to the scientific community.

Can a person be genetically predisposed toward homosexuality? Is an individual's sexual identity formed during the early stages of learning, in response to more-feminine or more-masculine role models? As in many other areas of psychology, the question of the origins of homosexuality — nature or nurture, genes or environment — remains a matter of speculation, as well as the subject of intense study and debate.

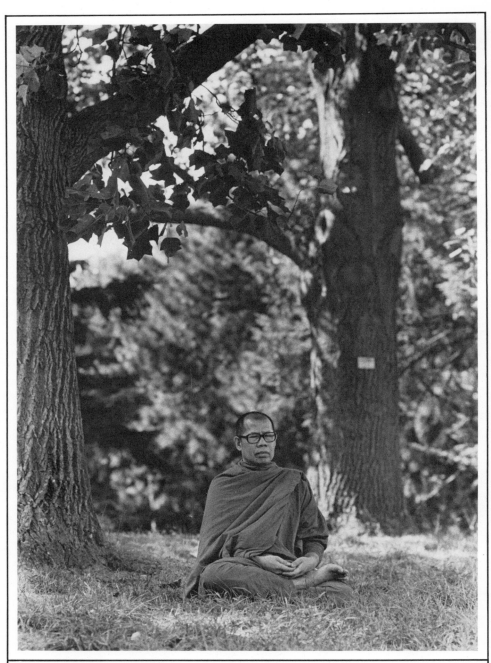

A man practices meditation, a healthy means of intentionally altering the way we perceive the world. Although drugs appear to offer relief from everyday troubles, they can be an unhealthy escape.

CHAPTER 8

ALTERED STATES OF CONSCIOUSNESS

The nature of consciousness may be the true final frontier of science. Sending a man to the moon is child's play compared to building a machine that can do what you do as you read this page. Indeed, there are many scientists who believe that no machine will ever have the ability to feel and think and be *aware* that it is doing so.

Yet with this ability to think there comes a burden as well, for consciousness brings with it the knowledge of one's own mortality, the knowledge of injustice and of cruelty. Because life's sad realities must be faced alongside its better half, there is the temptation to escape it all by simply altering the way we perceive the world around us. Sometimes the alteration occurs naturally, such as in sleeping and dreaming; it can also be brought about intentionally, as with hypnosis or meditation; and it can be induced chemically, with drugs used medically or recreationally. Drugs are used by many people wishing to alter their perceptions and, they think, reality. Though the problem remains that an "altered" state is as difficult to define as a "normal" state, the lesson here, as in the other books in this series, is that through the use of drugs it is usually only life's better side that is lost.

After all, consciousness as we know it did not happen by chance. It evolved over millions of years through a process called *natural selection*. In this process, all living organisms are shaped to best adapt to their environment. The emotions and thoughts that make up consciousness are two of the most essential tools that this process has given to human beings.

The Evolution of Consciousness

The nature of thoughts and emotions, and the connection between them, has always been a troublesome problem. In the brain's structure, however, scientists have discovered some interesting clues to this puzzle.

For many years, surgeons and psychologists have studied patients with wounds to the brain, so that today we have a fairly accurate map of how the parts of the brain affect behavior. This map suggests that the outer, upper layer of cells in the front part of the brain, the neocortex, is the brain's thought center, whereas a deeper, more central part of the brain, the limbic system, controls emotion.

The evidence for these conclusions is well established. First, it was discovered that a patient with a severe wound to the forehead will generally suffer a loss of reasoning ability but may still be able to display appropriate emotions; a wound to the limbic system, however, will often leave some thought processes intact, but result in inappropriate emotional responses. Sophisticated experiments involving electrical stimulation of these areas have borne out such behavioral findings, so that while much of the brain remains a mystery, we can at least safely say that we think with our neocortex, but feel with our limbic system.

If we combine this fact with the way the brain has evolved over millions of years, a fascinating story begins to emerge — a story not only about the difference between feeling and thinking, but about how and why we feel and think the way we do.

The first creatures to walk the earth, the dinosaurs, developed immense and complicated bodies, but never attained much in the way of brain power. They had what scientists today call a "reptilian" brain — hardly more than a small bundle of nerve cells — which enabled them to respond to the needs of hunger and thirst, avoid pain, and survive. Many animals today have no more than this primitive brain, but through millions of years of evolution a few species developed the next stage: the limbic brain.

This was a big step. The limbic brain, which was simply a growth of brain tissue around the earlier, more primitive brain of the reptiles, enabled an animal to feel true emotions rather than simply react to things. As a result, animals with this brain could display a much broader range of responses to their environment, and could adapt much more easily to changing conditions such as climate. But this was more than

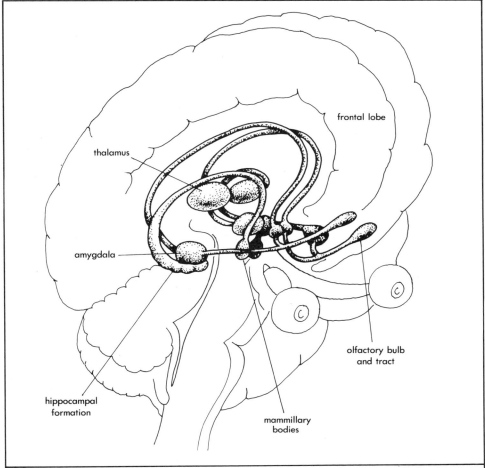

The limbic system controls emotions. An injury to this area of the brain will leave some thought processes intact but will often result in inappropriate emotional responses.

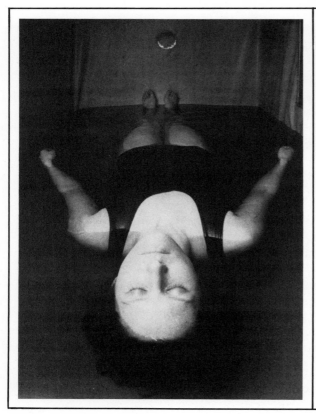

A woman lies in a sensory deprivation tank. Some people feel that once their outside perceptions are thus reduced, they can achieve a feeling of serenity or "inner peace."

a simple increase in complexity or efficiency. Imagine the behavior of a group of chimpanzees — the humanlike way that they frolic and tease each other — and then consider the lizard, with its mechanical, stop-and-go movements. This is the difference between the limbic and the reptilian brain.

The next step in the evolution of the brain produced the neocortex, which has been aptly called "nature's masterpiece." Unique to man, this dense layer of brain cells developed upward and forward from the older limbic brain to form the most complex and powerful information system on earth — thousands of times more powerful than the largest computer. It is the neocortex that gives human beings their sense of consciousness and control, permitting them to cope with life by planning deliberately and then acting accordingly. But most important, it is the neocortex that gives us language, and through language, thought.

The connection between thought and language may not be apparent at first. But consider the sentence you are reading right now; without language, how could you understand the thought that it is expressing? Without language, could you even ask yourself that question? The answer is that without language, all but the simplest forms of thought would be impossible, because the abilities to sense, to feel, to remember, and to learn from experience still do not add up to the ability to understand. Language acts like a net in which to hold our experiences, feelings, and memories, and, like a net, language can be used to capture things — in this case individual ideas, as opposed to vague feelings and emotions.

The development of the neocortex in humans thus enabled them to truly think, instead of simply feel and react. Nevertheless, the limbic brain still exists in modern man and woman, and still controls their emotions in ways that are not always rational. Even the reptilian brain, in the form of the brainstem, still exists in modern man and woman, and it, too, sometimes overrides both emotions and rationality. Thus, after millions of years of evolution, the individual remains part reactor, part feeler, and part thinker.

Naturally "Altered"

Sleeping and dreaming, the only naturally occuring "altered" states of consciousness, have been interpreted in many different ways. Freud considered the content of dreams to be

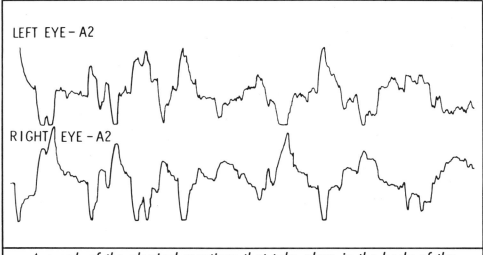

LEFT EYE – A2

RIGHT EYE – A2

A graph of the physical reactions that take place in the body of the sleeper during the rapid eye movement (REM) stage of sleep.

the repressed corners of the mind. Some more recent psychologists think that dreaming is not a process of repression but one of activation, the highlighting of the day's events. Another recent theory holds that the very purpose of dreaming is not to highlight certain events but to allow the mind to *forget* them once the dream is done. And a theory that incorporates parts of each of these first three theories would have it that dreams merely process the hidden or forgotten moments of recent experience.

The five stages of sleep, from dreaming to deep sleep, are altered states of consciousness that pervade each part of the evolving brain — reactor, feeler, and thinker — with a unique pattern of the use of our perceptual tools. But, interestingly, experiments done in the early 1970s showed that sleep deprivation, which can lead to hallucinations and paranoia, does not much hinder cognitive or learning functions if the person wants to perform them. In other words, the reasoning part of the brain, centered in the neocortex, seems not to require as much rest as the other parts. Indeed, if sleep *deprivation* is considered an altered state unto itself, and if learning is not much hindered by it, what might that say about the evolutionary role of the neocortex? It could be that human reason is one of our most resilient traits.

Seeking a Higher Perceptual Plane

We have little active control over our somnolent thoughts. But there are self-regulated altered states of consciousness under the category of meditation. In the 1960s and 1970s, transcendental meditation (TM) was one form of meditation that gained great popularity in this country. Such meditative techniques as yoga and Zen have been major components of Eastern philosophical and religious beliefs for centuries.

One purpose of meditation is to purify or cleanse the mind and body, and to elevate the psyche to a higher level of perceiving the world. Other forms of meditation are designed simply to help one relax and reduce stress.

It is fairly easy to practice meditation, and there are several ways of achieving a meditative state. First, you must be in quiet surroundings, free of distraction. You can either chant or repeat a certain sound or word (called a *mantra* by TM practitioners), regulate breathing, or not think of anything at all. If done properly and over a period of time, meditation can produce an aware yet relaxed state in which perceptions can be elevated beyond those of the ordinary waking state.

Physiologically, brain wave patterns change during meditation, often showing an increase in alpha waves, which are associated with relaxation. Additionally, respiration and heart rate, along with oxygen consumption, decrease in the meditative state, further slowing the metabolism and relaxing the body. Some experienced yogis have gone into such deep states of meditation that their brain wave patterns were not affected even when onlookers made noises next to the yogi's ear or placed a hot object on his skin.

Drugs and the Brain

We all use drugs, which may affect our personalities and lives either minimally or profoundly. We take aspirin for a headache, vitamins to supplement our diet, antibiotics when we are ill. These types of drugs, however, do not directly interact with the central nervous system, as psychoactive drugs do. Psychoactive drugs can have medical uses, but more commonly they are taken recreationally or out of addictive need. The direct, physical impact of drugs on the brain has been well studied, but the impact of drugs on human emotion is harder to trace — most brain studies are done on animals, and animals simply do not have the emotions that humans do.

Among the most common drugs is nicotine. According to the American Lung Association, "Cigarette smoking prematurely kills more people — some 350,000 annually — than heroin, cocaine, and other illicit drugs, plus automobile accidents, homicide, suicide, and alcohol abuse combined." Caffeine is also a prevalent drug, found chiefly in coffee, tea, soft drinks, and candy bars. Nicotine and caffeine are both stimulants, which means their chief effect is to speed up the central nervous system and many brain functions.

Alcohol, on the other hand, is a depressant, and can greatly alter normal mood and emotion. Used moderately, alcohol is socially acceptable and, for most people, relatively harmless. For the estimated 6 million Americans who are alcoholics, however, the drug can be devastating.

As a depressant, alcohol acts as a sort of brake on the brain. Under the influence of alcohol, one's alertness and motor coordination decrease, while reaction time is slowed.

Some researchers think that alcohol kills neurons all over the brain. Although it is likely that alcohol does directly cause some brain damage, it has not been possible to pinpoint specific levels of neuronal loss in various brain areas.

Some side effects or cofactors of alcoholism are also degenerative. A case in point is Korsakoff's syndrome. Patients with Korsakoff's syndrome display a profound loss in memory, and they respond to the memory loss in a unique way. Instead of saying "I can't recall," they confabulate, making up statements to cover up their memory loss. For many years physicians thought that Korsakoff's syndrome was due to a vitamin deficiency — especially of the B vitamins — that resulted from the poor diet of alcoholics. However, direct neuronal damage due to alcohol is probably of importance along with any vitamin deficiency.

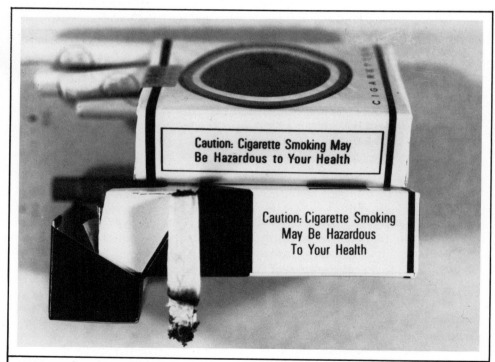

An early version of the mandatory warning that now appears on each pack of cigarettes. The drug compounds in cigarettes kill more people each year than all other drugs combined.

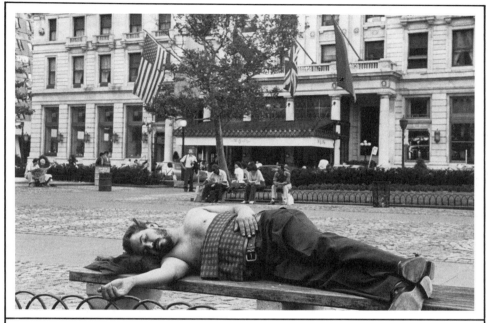

A street person sleeps on a bench in New York City. Many of the nation's homeless are victims of alcoholism.

Illegal Drugs

The destructive effects of alcohol, a legal psychoactive drug, are well documented. Other psychoactive drugs, particularly illegal narcotics such as heroin, and hallucinogens such as LSD (lysergic acid diethylamide) and PCP (phencyclidine), influence normal behavior in dramatic and often disastrous ways. LSD and PCP disrupt the brain's ability to effectively sort, organize, and interpret information. In many cases, users have experienced a total break with reality and suffered permanent psychological disorders.

LSD has the effect of mimicking a natural neurotransmitting chemical in the brain called serotonin, which plays a role in sensory perception. By overstimulating the brain's receptors for serotonin, LSD causes heightened sensations of some kinds, particularly visual and spatial. It also causes marked distortions of perception, and aberrations in an individual's sense of self. Under the influence of LSD, many men and women panic at the feeling that they are losing their personal identity. Some become psychotic. Others have jumped from windows of high buildings.

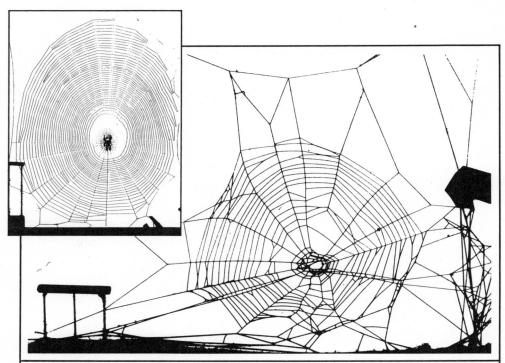

A normal spider's web (left) and a web spun while the spider was under the influence of phenobarbital. Drugs can impair even routine tasks and also have tragic effects on human users.

PCP, also known as "angel dust," has been known to cause severe psychotic reactions in which users experience a total break with reality. Some users have even killed friends or family members while under the influence of PCP and later said they had no idea what they had done.

Marijuana has a more complex chemical structure than most psychoactive drugs, and many of its compounds are toxic, including its smoke. Its harmful effects on the lungs and respiratory system are similar to those of cigarettes, but the psychoactive elements are harder to pin down. Regular use seems to have a cumulative effect, the real damage not appearing for some years. But a general deterioration of some intellectual and psychological functions has been reported in many long-term users; moreover, long-term abusers of marijuana have reported that certain cognitive and emotional problems that they experienced before their marijuana use began worsened during the period they used the drug.

Learning and Drugs

Drugs affect the learning process, usually for the worse. In laboratory experiments, it has been shown that performance is invariably altered when subjects are under the influence of drugs. The chemical substances distort reaction time, cognitive function, and even the ability to distinguish between reality and fantasy.

Some drugs seem initially to aid in the learning process. For example, in moderation, caffeine increases alertness and speeds reaction time. But too much caffeine will ultimately cause fatigue and anxiety, thereby decreasing performance.

Similarly, cocaine was once thought to be a wonder drug, and for a number of years earlier in this century was not only legal but was used as an ingredient in some wines, soft drinks, and over-the-counter elixirs. Rather than directly speeding up synaptic activity, cocaine interferes with natural brain substances that put a brake on excessive neurotransmission. The result, though, is overstimulation, leading to rapid and powerful addiction.

Alcohol and other depressants can greatly slow reaction time and reduce motor skills, so that a person who has been drinking and attempts to drive an automobile will show diminished performance. Nowhere is this fact more evident than in accident statistics. According to police records, alcohol is a contributing factor in fully half of all traffic deaths each year in the United States.

Drugs and Memory

Thanks to the increasing amount of research on Alzheimer's disease, which claims an estimated 100,000 lives each year, more and more evidence is being obtained linking the neurotransmitter acetylcholine with memory. As mentioned in Chapter 5, the brains of many Alzheimer's patients show a marked decrease of acetylcholine compared to those of healthy individuals. Moreover, when certain drugs, such as bethanechol, are used to boost acetylcholine levels, memory impairment in Alzheimer's patients is not as severe. Unfortunately, scientists have yet to discover a safe and consistently effective drug to restore acetylcholine to normal levels.

Although drugs such as alcohol, marijuana, cocaine, and LSD can cause temporary and even permanent memory damage, certain chemical substances like the acetylcholine restorers hold great promise for enhancing memory, not only in Alzheimer's patients but in the general population as well.

Several large drug companies, for example, are trying to synthesize a "memory pill," which would be available to stroke victims and Alzheimer's patients, and even healthy men and women who suffer mild memory loss. Like other bodily functions, memory does diminish with age (beginning at about the age of 30), so a memory pill could be of immense benefit to society—if it can do all that we hope it will.

Drug companies are not only targeting acetylcholine restorers in their research on memory but also other classes of drugs. One class is nootropics (from the Greek word *noos*, meaning "mind"). The prototype in this series, Piracetam, was not originally designed to enhance memory but rather to quell motion sickness. However, its positive effects on memory have prompted its Belgian manufacturer to market the drug in various parts of the world as an antigeriatric. According to some researchers, such memory-enhancing pills could be on the market for general use before the turn of the century.

Drug Use and Being "Normal"

Though the percentage has dropped slightly since the early 1980s, more than four-fifths of all teenagers have experimented with drugs of some sort — alcohol, marijuana, cocaine, amphetamines, or hallucinogens. But experimentation does not make a person normal or abnormal, just as abstinence from all drugs is not a sign of normality or abnormality. What is "normal" in one's group of friends is not necessarily normal or right for the individual, especially if it involves drug use.

Drug use, like other behavior, must be weighed in combination with a wide range of other behavior and thoughts. Even well-adjusted people are given to maladjusted behavior like cigarette smoking and occasional abnormal behavior like rage, depression, or extreme anxiety. Although human beings may strive for perfection in their lives, the idea of a perfect person or a perfect world is simply unrealistic. Perfection, if there was such a thing, would be the most abnormal behavior of all.

Yet it *is* normal to wish an occasional escape from a turbulent world. Escape, even in the form of daydreaming, is a method of coping with pain, anxiety, or fear when none of the primary joys such as love or comfort is readily attainable. And coping strategies, as mentioned, are part of the delicate balancing act that a healthy personality employs. It is when any one strategy — such as mental escape or sleep — begins to dominate a person's actions that the balance suffers. (Needless to say, drug use is never an effective or advisable coping strategy.) The precariously achieved "normal" state of general contentment, motivation, and emotional sensitivity is something the human brain is equipped to sustain. Too-frequent alteration of the natural state often begins as an experiment and ends as permanent or uncontrollable disruption.

As research on the brain progresses — and it is progressing rapidly as the 20th century nears its end — we move closer to understanding the key elements of human emotion and thought. But if there is one aspect of the universe that we are destined never to grasp fully, it may well be our own psychological makeup. Can the mind hold up a mirror to view itself from every angle?

Further Reading

Bylinsky, George. "Medicine's Next Marvel: The Memory Pill." *Fortune*, January 20, 1986, 68–71.

Calder, Nigel. *The Human Conspiracy: The New Science of Social Behavior*. New York: Viking Press, 1976.

Hall, Stephen S. "The Brain Branches Out." *Science*, June 1985, 72–74.

Long, Patricia. "Laugh and Be Well?" *Psychology Today*, October 1987, 28–29.

Maslow, Abraham H. *Toward a Psychology of Being*. New York: Van Nostrand Reinhold, 1968.

Petersen, Anne C. "Those Gangly Years." *Psychology Today*, September 1987, 28–34.

Restak, Richard M., M.D. *The Brain: The Last Frontier*. New York: Doubleday, 1979.

Rosen, Clare M. "The Eerie World of Reunited Twins." *Discover*, September 1987, 36–46.

Sartre, Jean-Paul. *The Emotions: Outline of a Theory*. New York: Philosophical Library, 1948.

Sheehan, David V., M.D. *The Anxiety Disease*. New York: Scribners, 1983.

Smith, Samuel. *Ideas of the Great Psychologists*. New York: Harper & Row, 1983.

Snyder, Solomon H., M.D. *The Troubled Mind: A Guide to Release from Distress*. New York: McGraw-Hill, 1976.

Travis, Carol. "Coping with Anxiety." *Science Digest*, February 1986, 46–50, 80–81.

Winokur, George, M.D. *Depression: The Facts*. New York: Oxford University Press, 1982.

Zinberg, Norman. *Alternate States of Consciousness*. New York: The Free Press, 1977.

Glossary

acetylcholine a chemical substance believed to be the body's major neurotransmitter, or chemical messenger; plays an important role in the transmission of nerve impulses, especially at synapses; centrally involved in the cognitive process of storing and retrieving information from memory

acupuncture a process in which certain specific tissues of the body are pricked with needles to relieve pain or anesthetize localized areas of the body

acute describing a condition in which the symptoms are often severe but short in duration

addiction a condition caused by repeated drug use, characterized by a compulsive urge to continue using the drug, a tendency to increase the dosage, and physiological and/or psychological dependence

AIDS Acquired Immune Deficiency Syndrome; an acquired defect in the immune system, thought to be caused by a virus (HIV) and spread by blood or sexual contact; leaves people vulnerable to certain infections and cancers that are often fatal

Alzheimer's disease an illness characterized by irreversible loss of memory, disorientation, possible problems with speaking or walking, and decline of intellectual abilities

androgen one of several principally male sex hormones; the main androgen is testosterone, which controls the development of male sex organs

anxiety an emotional state similar to stress and fear; caused by tension or distress, or the anticipation of tension or distress

behavioral conditioning any of a number of methods used to teach or reinforce specific types of behavior

chronic describing a long-term condition that may vary in intensity but is always present

cocaine the primary psychoactive ingredient in the coca plant and a behavioral stimulant

cognition the mental processes involved with rational thought, perception, and memory

compulsive behavior an uncontrollable action performed repeatedly

dendrite one of many branched extensions of a neuron that receives information from other neurons' axons at synaptic junctions and transmits it in electric form to the neuron's cell body and axon

depression a psychological state of varying intensity characterized by symptoms such as withdrawal, ennervation, unhappiness, helplessness, and hopelessness

endorphin a compound produced in the brain that serves as a natural opiate to the body

estrogen the principal female sex hormone, which controls the female reproductive functions and secondary sex characteristics

heroin a semisynthetic opiate produced by a chemical modification of morphine

hormone a chemical released into the bloodstream from endocrine glands such as the thyroid or pituitary gland; hormones travel throughout the body to activate receptors located on specific organs; they activate and/or regulate many bodily processes

hypothalamus a region at the base of the brain involved in the regulation of thirst, hunger, sex drive, and body temperature; also plays a vital role in governing the endocrine system and the emotions

limbic system a complex system of nerve pathways and networks in the brain, involving several different nuclei, that is involved in the expression of instinct and mood in activities of the endocrine and motor systems of the body, including self-preservation and preservation of the species; the expression of fear, rage, and pleasure; and the establishment of memory patterns

LSD lysergic acid diethylamide; a hallucinogen derived from the ergot fungus that grows on rye, or from morning glory seeds

maladaptive behavior actions that generally do not conform to accepted social standards and can indicate mental and physical disorders; all normally functioning individuals invariably exhibit maladaptive behavior on occasion, but this does not necessarily inhibit overall successful functioning in society

memory the faculty by which individuals process, store, and retrieve information from the brain

motivation a state brought on by a cognitive or biological need that prompts behavior

mnemonic device a memory-aiding system devised to help the mind reproduce an unfamiliar idea

nature-nurture an ongoing debate regarding whether heredity or environment shapes human behavior

neurotransmitter a chemical released by neurons that transmits nerve impulses across a synapse

nicotine an addictive, poisonous, psychoactive alkaloid found in tobacco

normal emotional behavior a term that encompasses a wide spectrum of behavior, which, at times, includes maladaptive and even abnormal behavior

opiate compound derived from the milky juice of the poppy plant *papaver somniferum*, including opium, morphine, codeine, and heroin

PCP phencyclidine (commonly known as angel dust), a hallucinogen originally developed as an anesthetic

perception the act of processing and interpreting sensory information to gain awareness and make judgments

phobia a continuing, extreme, and irrational fear

physical dependence adaption of the body to the presence of a drug such that its absence produces withdrawal symptoms

placebo a medicine that is pharmacologically ineffective but may help to relieve a condition because the patient believes it will; often used as a control in clinical trials of new drugs; often given to participants in psychological experiments

psychological dependence a condition in which the drug user craves a drug to maintain a sense of well-being and feels discomfort when deprived of it

schizophrenia a mental disorder in which a person loses touch with reality; characterized by profound emotional withdrawal and bizarre behavior, often including delusions and hallucinations

severe mental disorders any one of a number of extreme mental states characterized by a loss of contact with reality, a general deterioration of the personality, and often a loss of self-control

synapse the narrow gap between neurons, across which neurotransmitters pass to act on receptors

tolerance a decrease of susceptibility to the effects of a drug due to its continued administration, resulting in the user's need to increase the drug dosage in order to achieve the effects experienced previously

withdrawal the physiological and psychological effects of discontinued use of a drug

PICTURE CREDITS

Index

Bruce Friedland, a former reporter for the *Baltimore Sun* and editor for the Hearst Newspapers' *Baltimore News American*, is currently a technical publications editor for the Westinghouse Electric Corporation.

Joann Ellison Rodgers, M.S. (Columbia), became Deputy Director of Public Affairs and Director of Media Relations for the Johns Hopkins Medical Institutions in Baltimore, Maryland, in 1984 after 18 years as an award-winning science journalist and widely read columnist for the Hearst newspapers.

Solomon H. Snyder, M.D., is Distinguished Service Professor of Neuroscience, Pharmacology and Psychiatry at The Johns Hopkins University School of Medicine. He has served as president of the Society for Neuroscience and in 1978 received the Albert Lasker Award in Medical Research. He has authored *Uses of Marijuana, Madness and the Brain, The Troubled Mind, Biological Aspects of Mental Disorder,* and edited *Perspective in Neuropharmacology: A Tribute to Julius Axelrod.* Professor Snyder was a research associate with Dr. Axelrod at the National Institutes of Health.

Barry L. Jacobs, Ph.D., is currently a professor in the program of neuroscience at Princeton University. Professor Jacobs is author of *Serotonin Neurotransmission and Behavior* and *Hallucinogens: Neurochemical, Behavioral and Clinical Perspectives.* He has written many journal articles in the field of neuroscience and contributed numerous chapters to books on behavior and brain science. He has been a member of several panels of the National Institute of Mental Health.